THE CULTURAL CRISIS OF
MODERN MEDICINE

THE CULTURAL CRISIS
OF MODERN MEDICINE

EDITED BY JOHN EHRENREICH

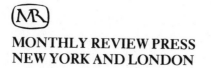

MONTHLY REVIEW PRESS
NEW YORK AND LONDON

Library of Congress Cataloging in Publication Data
Main entry under title:
The cultural crisis of modern medicine.
    Includes bibliographical references.
    1. Social medicine—Addresses, essays, lectures. 2. Medicine—
Political aspects—Addresses, essays, lectures. 3. Women's health
services—Addresses, essays, lectures. I. Ehrenreich, John, 1943–
RA418.C84   362.1'042   78-465
ISBN 0-85345-438-8

Monthly Review Press
62 West 14th Street, New York, N.Y. 10011
47 Red Lion Street, London WC1R 4PF

Manufactured in the United States of America

10 9 8 7 6 5 4 3 2 1

ACKNOWLEDGMENTS

This book started out as a joint venture with Barbara Ehrenreich. Due to the press of other work, Barbara had to withdraw from full participation in its preparation, but the overall concept of the book as well as many of the ideas developed in the introduction owe much to many discussions with her over the last few years.

Barbara and John Ehrenreich, "*Medicine and Social Control*," originally appeared in *Welfare in America: Controlling the Dangerous Classes*, ed. Betty Mandel (Englewood Cliffs, N.J.: Prentice-Hall, 1975), and in a shorter version in *Social Policy* (May-June 1974). Copyright © 1974 by Barbara and John Ehrenreich.

Irving Kenneth Zola, "Medicine as an Institution of Social Control," originally appeared in *Sociological Review* 20, no.4 (1972). Copyright © 1972 by *Sociological Review*, and reprinted by permission of the Editorial Board.

Marc Renaud, "On the Structural Constraints to State Intervention in Health," originally appeared in *International Journal of Health Services* 5, no.4 (1975). Copyright © 1976 by Baywood Publishing Company, Inc., and reprinted by permission.

Doris Haire, "The Cultural Warping of Childbirth," is an abridged version of an article that originally appeared in the International Childbirth Education Association *News* (Spring 1972). Copyright © 1972 by International Childbirth Education Association, and reprinted by permission.

Mary C. Howell, "Pediatricians and Mothers," is an edited version of a speech given to a conference on medical sociology at Temple University, Spring 1975. Reprinted by permission of the author. The poem, "I Like to Think of Harriet Tubman," if from Susan Griffin, *Like the Iris of an Eye* (New York: Harper & Row, 1976). Copyright © 1976 by Susan Griffin, and reprinted by permission.

Diana Scully and Pauline Bart, "A Funny Thing Happened on the Way to the Orifice: Women in Gynecology Textbooks," is an expanded version of an article that appeared in *American Journal of Sociology* 78, no.4 (January 1973). Copyright © 1973 by The University of Chicago.

CONTENTS

vii

THE CULTURAL CRISIS OF
MODERN MEDICINE

JOHN EHRENREICH

INTRODUCTION: THE CULTURAL CRISIS OF MODERN MEDICINE

Medical care is a good probe of the quality of a society. It reveals how a society deals with such fundamental individual and social experiences as birth and death, pain, disability, suffering, and aging. Viewed through the prism of its medical care system, the United States appears a very unhealthy society indeed. The twelve essays in this book, unlike most radical critiques of health care, are not concerned primarily with the problem of the distribution of health care (who gets what kind of care and how do they pay for it) but rather with the nature of modern medical care itself. They examine medical care as science and as social interaction. They ask what the real value of scientific medical care is—and what the price of that care is, in terms of physical harm, social dependency, and political impotence. In short, these are contributions to what we might call a "cultural critique" of modern medicine.

In this introductory essay I will discuss the historical and political origins and the principal themes of this "cultural critique." I will also examine its relation (which, we shall see, is partly complementary, partly antagonistic) to the political and economic critique of health care which radicals and socialists have more usually made. Finally, I will lay out some of the elements of a synthesis between the various radical approaches to health care to form a vision of what a truly socialist medicine might look like.

I want to thank Barbara Ehrenreich. Her ideas and criticisms contributed greatly to this essay.

1

THE RADICAL CRITIQUE OF MEDICAL CARE

To start with, let us recall the more traditional radical critique of medical care—what I will call the "political economic critique." (I should stress that in distinguishing this mode of criticism from the "cultural critique," which I shall come to shortly, I am deliberately exaggerating the gulf between the two for purposes of clarity. In actual practice, although pure forms of each critique are easy to identify, most radical critics of the health system draw elements from both.)

The political economic critique concentrates its fire on the inequitable distribution of health services. To the political economic critic, American medicine at its best is unquestionably beneficial. The problem is that not everyone has equal access to it. The poor are worst off, of course; they simply cannot afford good care (or, in some cases, any care at all). But finances are not the only barriers to care. Poor geographic distribution of doctors and hospitals (e.g., the lack of services in rural areas), lack of general practitioners and other primary care physicians in some areas, racism, etc. all act to deny many American access to acceptable medical care. These criticisms of medical care in the United States apply somewhat less strongly to other advanced capitalist countries (where systems of national health insurance—as in France, Germany, Japan—or national health services—as in England and Sweden—ease the financial burden), although even in these other countries, class and geographic differentials persist. But they apply with redoubled force to the poor countries of the world, where modern health services of any kind are virtually confined to the middle and upper classes in urban areas; the urban and rural poor are simply left to their own devices.

The political economic critique as we have described it so far is shared by liberal and radical critics alike. The two groups part company when it comes to explaining why the health system has been unable to provide readily accessible and affordable medical services for all, and what has to be done to correct the situation. Liberals tend to argue that the United States, at least, does not really have a health *system*; it has a "nonsystem," a fragmented,

uncoordinated mélange of private entrepreneur doctors, independent private and public hospitals, virtually unregulated nursing homes, etc., descended from an earlier era when the organization of health care mattered less because health care was not very effective anyway.[1] The problems would be solved, they argue, by creating an organized health care *system*—national health insurance to enable people to pay for care; government regulation of hospital construction and cost structures; government aid to health manpower training; government sponsored mechanisms to oversee the quality of care.

Radical political economic critics, by contrast, see the private ownership and control of medical and paramedical institutions as the root of the problem.[2] The privately practicing doctors, privately controlled hospitals and nursing homes, privately owned drug and insurance and medical supply companies, are "not in business for people's health," the radicals argue. As long as this situation exists, it remains impossible to plan and regulate the health system in the interests of equity and service. The solution, they assert, is a publicly owned and controlled health system, modeled, perhaps, after that of England or Sweden or after the more completely publicly owned and highly organized health system of the USSR and the European communist countries.[3] Some radicals would take the argument one step farther and say that as long as capitalism—with its private ownership and control of the means of production, distribution and finance—persists, so will the system of unequal incomes, unequal education, unequal health risks, and unequal health services. But as the English and Swedish experiences make clear, socialized medicine, even if imperfect, is possible in an otherwise capitalist country and is quite effective in reducing, if not eliminating, inequities.

The political economic critique, of course, acknowledges that there are problems with health care other than distribution. Services are all too often of low technical quality; doctors and hospital workers may discriminate among patients because of their race or class or nationality or sex; services are often bureaucratically organized and unnecessarily fragmented; and so on. But, and I emphasize this point, these are seen as blemishes, as problems with the *organization* of medical care, and not as intrin-

sic to the nature of medicine itself. Modern scientific medicine *per se*, from the political economic perspective, is seen as an unalloyed benefit to humanity; and the triumph of modern medical practice over every form of superstition and quackery is seen as one of the great technical advances that capitalism will pass on to its socialist successors.

In the last fifteen years or so, another mode of criticism of modern medicine, typified by the essays in this anthology, has emerged. Developing out of the often mutually isolated experience and analysis of several disparate groups, it has not generally been seen as a single critique of the health system. But the separate lines of criticism of medical care developed by militant black community groups, by feminists, by radical psychotherapists, and by health policy analysts concerned with the impact of modern medicine are related, and benefit from being considered together. I will call this synthesis of these criticisms the "cultural critique" of modern medicine.

The political economic critique challenges the poor distribution of an otherwise admirable service; the cultural critique disputes the value of the services themselves. It challenges the assertion, common to liberal and radical critics of the political economic school (as well as to the American Medical Association and the American Hospital Association), that Western-style medical care is effective, humane, and desirable. (The implications of this contention for the questions of distribution raised by the political economic critique are evident: why expand access to something that's no good? I shall have considerably more to say about this problem below.)

What I am calling a cultural critique first appeared in the area of mental health. Psychiatry is the weakest link in modern medical care. Its efficacy is quite low. H. J. Eysenck summed up a 1965 review of the literature on the effectiveness of psychotherapy: "The therapeutic effects of psychotherapy are small or nonexistent and do not in any demonstrable way increase the rate of recovery over that of a comparable group which receives no treatment at all."[4] Eysenck's conclusions have been disputed, but clear evidence for a positive effect of psychotherapy is still lacking. Even among other doctors, psychiatry has relatively low

prestige; and its endemic sectarianism has not made it any more convincing as a scientific discipline. More important, psychiatry is concerned not with clinically measurable somatic disfunctions, but with what is *socially defined* as abnormal or unacceptable behavior. (That this is so is aptly illustrated by R. D. Laing's description of a man "gibbering away on his knees, talking to someone who is not there." It is only because we accept the social definition of this activity as *praying* that we do not see him as *mad*.)⁵ Psychiatry unabashedly proclaims its right to make moral judgments. It is the branch of medicine which openly specializes in the *social control* of deviant behavior.

To many, the twentieth-century understanding of alcoholism, drug addiction, homosexuality, etc. as "illness," rather than as sin or crime, seems a triumph of humanity (and compared to eighteenth- and nineteenth-century attitudes, no doubt it is). Expanding access to mental health services became a major goal of medical and other social reformers. But in the 1960s, just as this goal seemed to become realizable (through the Federal Community Mental Health Act, Medicaid, etc.), more and more people—not least, many mental patients and ex-patients—began to question its desirability. The boundaries of the socially and sexually permissible were rapidly expanding. Psychiatry lagged far behind, continuing to define as "sick" (and therefore subject to psychiatric "treatment") what a growing portion of society viewed as normal. More and more young people experimented with self-induced states that were psychologically "abnormal" (produced by drugs, meditation, etc.). Psychiatrists insisted on diagnosing a wide range of behavior—from antiwar activity to black "rioting" to being a "hippy"—as psychotic. The very medical notion of psychosis became suspect, tinged with political and social judgments. Psychiatry stood exposed, not as a science and not as unequivocally benign, but simply as a mode of social control operating to preserve the social status quo. As Thomas Szasz commented in his influential book *The Myth of Mental Illness*:

> Therapeutic interventions have two faces; one is to heal the sick, the other is to control the wicked . . . Contemporary medical practices—

in all countries regardless of their political makeup—often consist of complicated combinations of treatment and social control . . . . Psychiatric diagnoses are stigmatizing labels, phrased to resemble medical diagnoses and applied to persons whose behavior annoys or offends others.[6]*

During the same period, the Black Liberation movement and other radical community movements began to develop a not dissimilar critique of somatic medicine. For one thing, black, Hispanic, and Asian communities in big cities in the United States repeatedly attacked the racism of the medical system. Both the health status of minority communities and the health care available to them were demonstrably worse than in white communities.[7] More important to the development of a cultural critique of medicine, the actual medical encounters of nonwhite patients with doctors and other health workers were frequently stained by, if not saturated with, racism. Numerous exposés documented widespread medical abuse of nonwhite patients (e.g., involuntary sterilizations, testing of drugs without the patient's knowledge, "dumping" patients from one hospital to another). Even more commonly, doctors and nurses displayed hostile or openly racist attitudes to nonwhite patients. Doctors, hospital administrators, and medical sociologists could not understand why blacks and members of other minority groups did not fully utilize preventive services; failed to communicate clearly with the doctors; did not follow doctors' orders (for use of medications, return visits). The obvious explanation—that the nonwhite patients saw in their contact with the generally white doctors not a technically neutral, personally benign encounter, but a hostile social interaction dominated by the doctor—was evident to the

---

* I do not mean to suggest that psychiatry has no therapeutic value under any circumstances, or that all mental disturbance is benign (either from the standpoint of the disturbed person or of society). The whole topic is clouded by the difficulties in defining what constitutes "neurotic" or "psychotic" behavior on the one hand and what constitutes a "cure" on the other. A full discussion is beyond the scope of this essay and this book, which are primarily concerned with a social analysis of *somatic* medicine. The significance of the attacks on psychiatry, for our purposes, is the insights that they provided into the entire medical endeavor.

nonwhite communities if not to the doctors. Like the schools and the welfare system, the medical system began to be perceived not as benevolent but as a system of social control. (The experience of nonwhite patients in the United States with white-dominated health services closely parallels the experience of Algerian patients with French colonial doctors and hospitals, graphically described by Frantz Fanon; see his article, "Medicine and Colonialism," in this volume.) Thus, intensified community struggles against racism forced attention onto the nonmedical aspects of the interpersonal relations involved in medical care.

The radical community movements also developed a growing skepticism about *professionalism*. Doctors and professional (registered) nurses had long insisted that professionalism was a mechanism for maintaining high standards of care and a commitment to social service. But by the mid-sixties, doctors and professional nurses had come to make up only a minority of the people actually delivering health care. The rapid expansion and growing technical complexity of medical services required an explosive growth in the number of nonprofessional health workers—nurses aides, orderlies, ward clerks, therapy aides, community health and mental health aides, and so on. Many of these workers were drawn from the black and other nonwhite communities. They rapidly came into conflict with the doctors and professional nurses. For one thing, they were strategically placed to observe the actual behavior of doctors and nurses and to compare it to the latter groups' self-proclaimed mission of service and compassion. Moreover, in their role as workers, they discovered professionalism was often a defense of occupational and class privilege rather than of high standards. For example, in and out of the hospital, nonprofessional health workers found that it was all but impossible to gain access to professional jobs, which offered higher pay, higher status, and greater opportunities to use their abilities and insights fully. Access to these jobs required passing through an educational gauntlet, set up by the organizations of the (largely white) professionals (the American Medical Association, American Nurses Association, etc.). And the skills and standards imposed by this educational process often seemed arbitrary, determined more by the professionals' desire to limit access

to their occupation (and to insure that only those meeting certain social and cultural standards be so much as eligible) than by any real concern with competency or desire to provide service.[8]

Not only workers, but also community groups became skeptical about professionalism. Seeking a greater say in how community medical institutions (e.g., hospital emergency rooms and clinics) ran, they found doctors using professionalism to defend their administrative powers. "Next they'll try to tell us how to operate," was the common response to community demands such as more convenient clinic hours and bilingual personnel in Hispanic communities. The doctors and nurses might proclaim professionalism to be a defense of high standards. But to nonprofessional workers and community groups it looked a lot more like a defense of power and privilege against the needs of other health workers and the community.

The growing realization that the "emperor has no clothes" did not long remain abstract. In 1968 in a state hospital in Topeka, and a year later in New York's Lincoln Hospital, nonprofessional hospital workers and their allies in the neighboring communities seized control of parts of hospitals and, with the aid of a few young radical doctors and other health professionals, operated certain services themselves. In 1970 in New York, the Young Lords, a radical Puerto Rican organization, "liberated" and operated a mobile x-ray unit and organized medical students and nonprofessionals to screen residents of the Barrio for lead poisoning, anemia, etc. In Chicago, San Francisco, and other cities, radical medical students, nonprofessionals, and a handful of sympathetic doctors operated free clinics in which traditional professional decorum and the traditional division of labor were all but ignored. (For example, in one clinic in Minneapolis, patients were taught to perform their own clinical lab tests; and patients were encouraged to ask questions and talk with doctors as social equals.) The message was clear: possession of professional *skills* did not have to imply a *socially* unequal relationship between doctor, patient, and nonprofessional health worker.[9]

Close on the heels of the radical community movements emerged the Women's Liberation movement. Just as the black movement exposed the racism at the heart of the healing rela-

tion, so the feminist movement revealed its endemic sexism.[10] The unusual aspect of the Women's Liberation movement, from our perspective, is that through it the walls of individual privacy which normally characterize doctor-patient relationships were breached. Women talked to each other and wrote about what actually goes on between a doctor and his patient, a subject heretofore discussed only in the doctors' own biased reports and sociologists' indirect analyses. What was revealed were the countless ways in which doctors acted, in the guise of a medical relationship, to reinforce male domination: female patients (who, I might note, account for some 58 percent of all visits to doctors in the United States made by adults on their own behalf, plus many more visits as the supervisors of their children's health care) were put down, made to feel bad about their bodies, fed masses of misinformation about "proper" female anatomy, sexuality, personality, child-rearing practices, denied control of their own reproductive functions (through access to contraception and abortion), and more. (See the articles by Barbara Ehrenreich and Deirdre English, Diana Scully and Pauline Bart, Mary Howell, and Linda Gordon in this volume.)

The Women's Liberation movement also began to open up the previously taboo subject of the actual technical competency of doctors and of modern medicine altogether. Doctors' practice, it soon became evident, was governed as often by myth as by science. Doctors exhibited massive ignorance on such subjects as menstruation, birth control, menopause, breast-feeding, the proper management of childbirth, vaginal infections, the dangers of hormones (e.g., birth control pills, synthetic estrogens for postmenopausal women), and the dangers of x-rays (e.g., mammography). Sometimes the doctors' ignorance was fairly harmless; other times—for example, with respect to "the pill" and to the management of childbirth (see Doris Haire's article, this volume)—it was less benign; but in any case, it made the doctors' facade of expertise all the more oppressive.

As in the case of nonwhite communities, understanding led to (or sometimes came from) action. Women—individually and in groups—sought to regain control of medical technology for themselves, so that it could be developed and used in their own

interests rather than in the interests of doctors' or of the broader male-dominated society. For some, this meant pushing for a greater number of women in medical school. For others, it meant learning as much as they could about their bodies so as to be better able to challenge the doctors or do without them. (Thus the phenomenal popularity of the Boston Women's Health Collective's *Our Bodies, Our Selves*.) Still others developed new modes of delivery of services (e.g., gynecological self-help, in which women learned to examine and treat themselves or each other for pregnancy, vaginal infections, etc.) and new technologies (e.g., menstrual extraction, in which the menstrual fluid is removed by aspiration in a few minutes rather than through the usual physiological process of menstruation). And some (reinforced, perhaps, by the general antitechnological sentiment common to many feminists and to the sixties counterculture) reopened the exploration of premodern modes of healing—herbal remedies, massage, diet, etc. Counter to prevailing medical opinion, which saw these modes of healing as quackery and superstition, experience suggested that at least some of these methods worked as well as or better than "modern, scientific" medicine.

The final source of the cultural critique of modern medicine was from health analysts from a wide range of political perspectives, who observed that despite the fact that the United States spent more *per capita* on health care (both absolutely and relative to income) than any other nation, the indicators of health status suggested that we had far from the most healthy people in the world. Worse, annual health care expenditures were rising by tens of billions of dollars every year, yet it was hard to see any result in the form of improved health. The earlier part of the twentieth century had seen both dramatic improvements in medical knowledge and technology (e.g., immunizations, antibiotics, open-heart surgery, insulin therapy) *and* significant gains in longevity, infant survival rates, and other indicators of health. The conclusion that the improvements in medicine were responsible for the improvements in health was all but inescapable. But though the medical miracles continued to appear with regularity, and though expenditures on health doubled and redoubled, from

the mid-fifties on, gains in health were not so easy to come by: the indicators of health status showed little if any change (see accompanying table).*

Indicators of Health Status

	1920	1940	1955	1970
Infant mortality rate[a]	85.8	47.0	26.4	20.0
Male life expectancy at birth[b]	53.6	60.8	66.7	67.1
Female life expectancy at birth[b]	54.6	65.2	72.8	74.8
Male life expectancy, age 40[b]	29.9	30.0	31.7	31.9
Female life expectancy, age 40[b]	30.9	33.3	36.7	38.3
Personal health care expenditures (billion dollars/year)	n.a.	3.5	15.2	60.1

[a] Deaths, per 1000 live births, in first year of life
[b] Years

Sources: U.S. Bureau of Census, *Statistical Abstract of the United States, 1975* (Washington, 1975); United States Bureau of Census, *Historical Statistics of the United States, Colonial Times to 1957* (Washington, 1960); Herbert Somers, "Health Care Costs," in Boisfeuillet Jones, ed., *The Health of Americans* (New York, 1970).

Indeed, chronic and degenerative diseases such as heart disease and cancer, which affect primarily older people, had reached epidemic proportion. One result: in the two decades between 1950 and 1970—while health-care expenditures in-

---

* Indicators such as life expectancy are, of course, very crude indicators of how healthy a people are. If, for example, people's lives were freer of pain, though their longevity was no greater than in earlier centuries, we would properly conclude that their health had improved though their life expectancy had not. There does not, however, seem to be any compelling evidence that this is in fact what was happening in the fifties and sixties. (See Powles, "On the Limitations of Modern Medicine," p. 3).[11]

creased by $50 billion and the Medicare program dramatically expanded health-care opportunities for the elderly—male life expectancy at age sixty-five increased by just four months (from 12.8 years to 13.1 years)!

A growing disillusionment with the effectiveness of medical care led analysts to reexamine the presumed connection between earlier improvements in health and medical care. As early as 1959, microbiologist René Dubos had pointed out that most of the decline in the death rate from tuberculosis (the major killer of the nineteenth century in Western Europe and the United States) had *preceded* the availability of medical technology which could have had any impact on the disease. Dubos argued that factors other than medical care—e.g., better nutrition—must account for the improvement in health which the decline in tuberculosis implied. Thomas McKeown has dramatically extended Dubos' insight: McKeown examined the cause of the decline in deaths from a group of diseases whose disappearance as major killers accounts for the bulk of the decline in the overall death rate in England since the early nineteenth century (tuberculosis, scarlet fever, typhoid, typhus, cholera, diarrhea and dysentery, and smallpox). He concluded that the reasons for their disappearance as major causes of death were, in order of importance: first, improvements in the standard of living (e.g., nutrition, housing); second, improvements in control of the environment (e.g., water supply and other sanitary services); and only *third*, personal medical care. John Powles and A. L. Cochrane have summarized further evidence that the death rates for a number of major noninfectious diseases (e.g., cancer, heart disease) have not responded to modern medical approaches. Echoing the contentions of some feminists who charged that scientific medicine had been overrated, these studies suggested that modern medical care was and is, at best, much less effective at reducing morbidity and mortality than the doctors have claimed and most people have believed.[11]

Dubos, Hans Selye, and a number of other analysts suggested that part of the limitation of modern medicine lay in the approach to the causes and treatment of disease characteristic of Western medicine since the late nineteenth century (see Marc

Renaud, this volume). Modern Western medicine has been largely based on: (a) the doctrine of specific etiology: each disease is caused by a specific cause; if the cause (e.g., a germ) is present, the person will get the disease, if it is not, he or she will not; and (b) the machine model of the body: the body is conceived of as a machine, made up of a group of interacting physical (and chemical) parts; the functioning of these parts is independent of the mind of the organism. These doctrines have provided the underpinnings for much of the advance of scientific medicine. However, their limitations, even in dealing with infectious disease, have become more and more evident. Dubos, Selye, and others have stressed a multiple-cause model of disease, in which body, mind, and environment (including, but not limited to, exogenous microorganisms) *interact* to produce disease or to cure it; they have called for the reexploration of more holistic approaches to health and disease.[12]

These suggestions found sympathetic ears in the movements of the sixties. The black movement was stressing the socioeconomic roots of the poor health of their community—poor housing, poor nutrition, high levels of pollution, tremendous stress, and so on. The environmental movement was uncovering and publicizing the role of air and water pollution in causing disease; the occupational health movement (e.g., the Black Lung movement among coal miners) was doing the same for health and safety hazards on the job. And the counterculture was rediscovering the supposed health benefits of vegetarian diets, stress-reducing techniques, etc., while exploring ancient—often Oriental—health doctrines which take a more holistic view of disease processes.*

---

* The illogic of the conventional modern medical approach to contemporary problems of disease nowhere appeared so clear as with respect to cancer. Hundreds of millions of dollars a year are spent on the search for the biological mechanisms of carcinogenesis and tumor growth and for curative techniques. The patient diagnosed with cancer faces, at best, devastating courses of radiation or drug therapy or debilitating radical surgery. And yet, it is widely known that some 80 percent to 90 percent of all cancers are caused by largely avoidable environmental hazards—air pollution, smoking, food additives, pesticides, radiation, etc. Scientific medicine, for all its insights into the molecular mechanisms of carcinogenesis, has simply become unhinged from any fundamentally effective approach to the disease.

Critics of medicine such as Dubos were simply arguing that medicine was less powerful than it had claimed to be. But a further stream of criticism argued that modern medicine was both physically and socially *harmful*. The dangers of supposedly safe medications had been publicized in the early 1960s in cases such as the Thalidomide tragedy. But it was the feminists' exposure of the dangers of oral contraceptives in the late sixties that made this a continuing concern to a mass audience.[13] Soon information was accumulating on the prevalence of unnecessary (and often risky) surgery, on doctors' over-readiness to prescribe inappropriate or dangerous drugs, on overuse of dangerous diagnostic procedures, and more. Ivan Illich dramatically summed up the wide extent and devastating impact of such "iatrogenic disease" (disease produced by diagnostic or therapeutic procedures):

> The medical establishment has become a major threat to health . . . The pain, dysfunction, disability, and anguish resulting from technical medical intervention now rival the morbidity due to traffic and industrial accidents and even war-related activity, and make the impact of medicine one of the most rapidly spreading epidemics of our time.[14]

The actual harm done by medicine is not limited to physical disability, argues Illich, nor are harmful diagnostic and treatment procedures the only sources of medical injury. The entire social organization of medical care conspires to produce ill health: medical bureaucracies "create ill health by increasing stress"; suffering of all kinds becomes "hospitalized" while our homes become "inhospitable to birth, sickness, and death"; and people become increasingly dependent on the support of the organized medical system to the point where they are unable to deal themselves with their own bodily and spiritual needs. Indeed, he continues, "suffering, mourning and healing outside the patient role are labeled a form of deviance."[15] To Illich, then, medicine has become a major form of *social control*, drawing to its bosom a greater and greater part of the critical events of life and managing our responses to them. Regardless of whether it manages them well or badly, in the end it reduces our own ability to handle our own lives: it produces dependent, helpless people. The conclu-

sion that an increasing array of individual and social problems had become "medicalized" (i.e., had come to be seen as problems which the medical system could and should handle) was also reached by Irving Zola (see his article, this volume) and by Barbara Ehrenreich and myself (see her article, this volume). Zola suggested that the impact of the medicalization of social issues was to "depoliticize" them—to make problems stemming from social causes appear instead to be individual deviancy, solvable (or at least controllable) by the individual's doctor. Barbara Ehrenreich's and my own concern grew directly out of the questions about the doctor-patient relationship raised by the black and feminist movements. What is the impact, we asked, of a system which throws women, blacks, working-class people into intimate and complete dependency on white, male, upper-middle and upper-class doctors? The relationship, we suggested, is a powerful mechanism producing acquiescence in the overall social structure and its values.

We can now sum up the principal contentions of the cultural critique of modern medicine: modern medical care, contrary to the assumptions of the more traditionally radical political economy critique, does not consist of the administration by doctors of a group of morally neutral, essentially benign and effective techniques for curing disease and reducing pain and suffering. The techniques themselves are frequently useless and all too often actually physically harmful. The "scientific" knowledge of the doctors is sometimes not knowledge at all, but rather social messages (e.g., about the proper behavior of women) wrapped up in technical language. And above all, both the doctor-patient relationship and the entire structure of medical services are not mere technical relationships, but social relationships which express and reinforce (often in subtle ways) the social relations of the larger society: e.g., class, racial, sexual, and age hierarchy; individual isolation and passivity; and dependency on the social order itself in the resolution of both individual and social problems. (These characteristics of medicine are exhibited in almost caricature form in the imperialist uses of medicine—see the essays by James Paul, E. Richard Brown, Howard Levy, and Frantz Fanon in Part 3 of this book. As Marx commented, in writing of

the relevance of the relatively clearly developed social relations of 1860s England for more backward regions where capitalist relations were not so obvious, "Of you the story is told.") The assumption made in the political economic critique—that modern medicine, distributed through an equitable delivery system, would be enthusiastically embraced by a socialist society—is thus thrown into question. At its very core, asserts the cultural critique, medicine as we now know it is a capitalist mode of healing. What *parts* of it can be taken over into socialism is quite uncertain.

THE LIMITATIONS OF THE RADICAL CRITIQUE

I have described the major directions taken by radical criticism of the health system in recent years. Both the political economy critics and what I have called the "cultural" critics make compelling criticisms of contemporary medical care. But a word on their limitations is in order.

The political economic critique follows the conventional Marxist pattern of analysis: medical care is treated as a commodity like any other; the important things about medical care can then be derived from the general laws for the production and distribution of commodities. (Of course, in the case of medical care and other services, production and distribution occur simultaneously.) The primary problems that the political economic critic identifies by this analytic approach, then, are distributional: poor and working-class people in the United States and elsewhere do not have access to adequate care. By contrast, in a socialist society, health care would be socialized and everyone would have equal access to high quality care.

But medical care as we know it—i.e., as it has developed in capitalist society—is not just an unambiguously useful commodity like asparagus or shoes or swimming lessons. Like many other more complex commodities, it is thoroughly permeated with capitalist priorities and capitalist social relations. Not merely the distribution, not merely the transaction between doctor and patient, but the medical technology itself (which is based on certain assumptions about the nature of disease processes, the causation

and cure of disease, the relations of individuals to their own bodies and to social processes) embodies the social relations created by capitalistic society. It is by no means clear that we want to pass *these* along to socialist society; i.e., *socialized* medicine is not necessarily *socialist* medicine.

Medicine is not unique in this respect, of course. There are many other cases in which apparently neutral and objective technology is in fact penetrated by and helps recreate the social relations of the society which developed it: the single family housing unit presupposes (and creates) a noncollective mode of living; individual automobiles imply an entire conception of use of energy, use of time, and spatial organization of society; assembly line production techniques and machinery assume and reinforce the separation and antagonistic relation between mental and manual labor; and so forth. In medicine it is not quite so evident that this is the case. For one thing, an unusual amount of mystery surrounds the technology (the result, in part, of doctors' efforts to keep their knowledge esoteric); for another, the presumably benevolent purposes of the medical endeavor provide an unusually opaque disguise for the sometimes antagonistic social relations built into it.

The political economic critique, however, also seems to me to overemphasize the commodity-like nature of medical care altogether. The healing relation is not simply a commercial transaction. It is also a *direct* social relation between two people (usually of sharply differing class or sex or race), unmediated by the commodity form. The doctor is actually in there, touching and penetrating your body, asking intimate personal questions, giving you orders to follow at your life's peril, sympathizing and caring or scorning and disparaging. To more than one political economic critic—for whom only those matters stemming directly from relations of production are real, material, and worthy of respect—the personal interactions which go on in the doctor's office are unmaterialist, of no interest. This seems to me an extraordinary example of what Marx called the "fetishism of commodities," in which relations between people appear in the guise of relations between the products of their labor. To be sure, one aspect of the relation between doctor and patient is a com-

modity relationship—the doctor as producer and seller of the commodity of medical care, the patient as purchaser and consumer. But simultaneously, it is a direct relationship of personal support, of domination—even, in some cases, of physical exploitation. It is hard to see how much more "material" you can get than this. Marx's and Engels' comment in *The German Ideology* reminds us that a materialist analysis involves more than "economic" activities:

> We must begin by stating the first premise of all human existence, and therefore of all history, the premise namely that men must be in a position to live in order to be able to "make history." But life involves before everything else eating and drinking, a habitation, clothing, and many other things [including, presumably, care of the sick or disabled—ed.] . . . The production of life . . . appears as a double relationship: on the one hand as a natural, on the other hand as a social relationship.[16]

That social relations are contained in medical technology and in the healing relationship is far from a matter of purely academic interest. Understanding those social relations is the key to understanding how medicine, as it has gained in technical mastery over bodily processes, has lost its ties to people's daily mode of life, to their individual and social feelings about birth, death, suffering, pain and dependency. And this, in turn, helps us to understand such contemporary phenomena as the decline in faith in medicine; the continued influence of premodern healing modalities; the investing of supposedly technical medical questions—such as the effectiveness of Laetrile—with major political content; and the spread of "neurotic" dependency on the medical system with consequently soaring utilization and soaring expenditures.

The cultural critique thus has major political implications for health policy. The question raised by conservatives—why should we go on pouring money into health care when the only result is a rise in utilization of medical services without corresponding improvements in health?—is a reasonable question. Within the narrow political economic framework, however radical, it is unanswerable. Conversely, the lack of mass popular support for the various proposals for national health insurance or for bureau-

cratic forms of socialized medicine reflects the unarticulated understanding that there is something very wrong with medicine as we have come to practice it.

The political economic critique, of course, emerges out of a consciousness of scarcity and so it is less concerned about the nature of medical services than about their existence at all. The cultural critique, by contrast, emerges out of consciousness of plenty. It should not be thought, however, that it is thereby irrelevant to the poor nations of the world or to the needs of poor people in the rich countries. It may be true that it is only when we have the luxury of plenty that we can, for the first time, examine closely just what it is that we have plenty of. But the insights that the cultural critique has reached about medical care, if not the conditions under which it reached them, are highly significant for medical care in any society.

To give an analogy: it is primarily in the more affluent, industrialized countries that the knowledge, resources, and industrial need for new technological developments generate the rapid advance of science and technology. It goes virtually without saying that we expect the poor countries of the world to want and to use the scientific and technical insights developed under the conditions of the wealthy countries (including, often, the insight that technologies installed in the rich countries only a very few years ago may already be obsolete or otherwise faulty and should not be imitated, if possible). Ironically, the matter somehow seems more problematic when it comes to insights directly affecting human health and safety, such as the recent concern in the affluent countries over the dangers of industrial pollution, of nuclear power plants, of unsafe occupational conditions. In these cases, concern for overall development understandably comes first; but the very low priority often given to the insights on the potential *adverse* impacts of industrialization, the lack of significance ascribed to the dialectical relationship between the achievements and the tragic failures of the rich countries, is disturbing. The lesson that advanced capitalism teaches so clearly—that human well-being can not be guaranteed by industrialization—is certainly not the least important lesson to be learned from the affluent countries.

Returning to the case of medical care, the cultural critique's

concern for the overall efficacy, safety, and social impact of Western-style scientific medicine has wide application—to the poor as well as to the more affluent, to the industrialized socialist countries as well as to the industrialized capitalist countries, to the developing nations and to the developed. In fact, the cultural critique developed in the affluent West drew in part on the parallel approaches to medical care taken by the decidedly nonaffluent Chinese. Especially during and since the Cultural Revolution of 1966-1969, the Chinese health-care system has embraced many of the policies advocated by cultural critics of the United States and England—policies such as the radical deprofessionalization of medical care (e.g., barefoot doctors, shortened academic training of doctors); promotion of egalitarian relations between doctors and patients and other health workers; integration of holistic, traditional modes of medicine with Western modes; involvement of patients as active participants in their own cures; and concern with the social and political roots of disease.[17]* Many aspects of these policies stem from broader social and political concerns rather than from analysis of the problems of medical care *per se*, of course. But, as I shall discuss below, as soon as the assumption that medical care is merely a commodity is rejected, the fusion of questions of health policy and of overall political and social values is exposed.

The various critiques of scientific medicine which I have grouped together as the "cultural critique" are not *uniformly* applicable to nonaffluent situations, however. Far from it: parts of the cultural critique, in their extreme formulations at least, show clearly their origins in what the Chinese would call a "fat" country, and exhibit a serious lack of concern about the situation of scarcity which characterizes medical care for most of the world (and for a not inconsiderable part of the United States as well).

---

* Whether any of these policies stem from a Chinese analysis of Western medical experience (other than in its imperialistic form in pre-Liberation China) is questionable. Western concerns with the social impact of air pollution and of occupational health hazards do not appear to have found much echo in China. (Environmental concerns exist, but seem more aroused by problems of waste and efficiency than by potential health problems.)

Taking an obvious example, when Ivan Illich insists that "A world of optimal and widespread health is obviously a world of minimal and only occasional medical intervention,"[18] from the perspective of those who now have "minimal and only occasional medical intervention" he has "obviously" overstated the case against modern medicine to the point of vitiating the entire cultural critique.

Modern medicine does work, does prevent death and reduce pain and suffering, even if less often and less effectively than its admirers have claimed. For example, in a 1968 National Academy of Sciences study of the impact of prenatal and postnatal care on infant birth weight and infant mortality, women were classified according to their ethnic group; according to medical and social criteria indicating whether their babies were at high risk (e.g., a tubercular mother or a mother living in a slum area would be placed in the high risk category); and according to the adequacy of the medical care they received. In every risk group and every ethnic group, the more adequate the medical care, the more likely a favorable outcome (i.e., a healthy baby). Among low-risk mothers, improvements in medical care above a certain fairly low level had relatively little effect; but among higher risk mothers, every increment in medical care markedly improved the baby's chances of survival. Other studies have come to similar conclusions: statistically, at least, above a relatively modest level of medical care services, the marginal impact of additional medical services is low. But below that level of services, the reverse is true: providing medical services, even in the absence of changes in environment, housing, nutrition, and so on, produces significant improvements in health.[19] And, of course, numerous clinical trials and much clinical experience provide evidence for the beneficial impact of medical care in the case of particular diseases in individuals.

How, then, can we explain the overall failure of health to respond to additional inputs of medical care, as charged by Illich, Powles, and other cultural critics? We may, of course, simply be using inappropriate measures of health status.[20] More likely , the losses to health resulting from the combination of incompetent medical practice, poor distribution and low accessibility of ser-

vices, poor patient compliance with doctors' instructions, grow-ing environmental hazards, and clinical iatrogenesis (exaggerated by inappropriate and excessive uses of technology) balance off the gains in health produced by medical intervention. But not all of the negative influences on health are intrinsically associated with the United States' mode of medical practice. The cultural critique has properly identified causes of health and disease, both outside the purview and concerns and powers of modern medicine and within medical practice itself. But, seen from the perspective of those who now do not have access to modern medicine (the majority of the world's people), it has not made a case for eliminating most of medicine altogether.

Cultural critics, as we have seen, have also denounced medicine as a mode of extending bourgeois cultural and political hegemony. Medicine, they argue, produces dependency and re-duces individual autonomy; it reinforces racism and sexism; it depoliticizes a variety of social (class, race, gender) issues in such a way as to make them seem like individual problems. In sum, it is a major instrument of bourgeois domination. All of these con-cerns seem to me to be relevant not only to our own situation but also to people presently lacking care as they seek access to medi-cal services or seek to construct new health systems. But as was the case with the critique of the curing capacity of medical care *per se*, legitimate concern all too quickly can become one-sided. Medicine does have these impacts, among others, but in describ-ing how medicine shapes culture, it is easy to fall prey to a kind of elitest snobbery: culture appears as something which is simply "laid on" a passive, helpless mass. But the complex dialectical interplay between fundamental needs and manipulated needs, between the need for dependency and the need for autonomy on the part of patients, between benevolence and domination and greed on the part of doctors and health institutions, needs dissec-tion, not mere denunciation. The dependency and passivity characteristic of modern medical care are sought by patients as well as imposed by doctors; they reflect not only the interests of the doctors and of giant corporations, but also the needs of patients. Medicine as practiced in the United States may rein-

force dependency and passivity in the face of bourgeois domination; it does not, however, *create* them.

TOWARD A SOCIALIST HEALTH POLICY

The two modes of radical criticism of medical care—the political economic critique and the cultural critique—appear to be at least partly incompatible: the political economic critique is based on the assumption that modern medical care is worth having and struggling for, the very assumption that the cultural critique denies. The incompatibility between the two seems especially evident when medical services are cut back. With assaults on social services of all kinds the order of the day in the industrialized countries, restoration of the services available a few years ago seems highly desirable. But the cultural critique, with its stress on the limits of modern medicine, seems to play right into the hands of conservatives. To policy makers looking for justifications for continuing cutbacks in health services or trying to resist popular pressures for comprehensive (and expensive) national health insurance programs, the cultural critique provides a certain "liberal" legitimacy. (It is, of course, the part of the cultural critique which insists upon the uselessness of medical care that they seize upon; fiscal conservatives have not, to my knowledge, argued that health services should not be extended because they are inherently racist and sexist, or because they help preserve and legitimate the status quo!)

Conversely, hard times have led many liberals and radicals to reject the cultural critique entirely. It seems to them self-evident that the perception of scarcity, not the dangers of plenty, is the sense of grievance out of which a movement to demand the restoration and expansion of social services can come. Some even go so far as to drop the more radical versions of the political economic critique as politically impractical; they replace, for instance, the demand for a national health service with the demand for a national health insurance system (i.e., a system to finance care, which would remain privately delivered and controlled).[21] Others preserve parts of the cultural critique, but only

nominally: they relegate changes in the nature of health care and the meaning of health to some far-off postrevolutionary period, when the class control of health institutions will have changed; for all present and practical purposes, they limit their demands to those flowing out of the political economic critique.[22]

But to limit the critique of medicine to complaints about its scarcity is to surrender the insights gained in the last few years; it is to say that despite the powerful critique of medical care developed in the last decade, we will take any crumbs that they will give us. This, of course, is precisely one of the "purposes" of cutbacks and recession in capitalist society: to make people satisfied with, even grateful for, much less than they had come to expect and demand.

The dilemma is a familiar one in Left history, of course. On the one hand, a "cultural critique" of existing institutions seems irrelevant in the face of existing scarcity. The tendency is to put it off until some affluent, postrevolutionary and "post-scarcity" period. On the other hand, struggling around the distribution of commodites, when the demand for these commodities and the commodities themselves have been hideously deformed by bourgeois social relations, risks falling into the narrowest, most limited reformism. "Reform or revolution"—upon the pole of this dichotomy the Left has been stuck for more than half a century.

How can we escape this dilemma? How do we build a movement that can go from what we have to what is implied by the full radical critique of medical care, given that even what we have now is endangered? Much of the argument between proponents of the two modes of critique seems to me sterile, unable to provide insight into this question. To develop a socialist health policy we must create a dialectical understanding of the crisis in medical care which draws from and integrates both political economic and cultural concerns.

To start with, we must reject the belief that the two approaches to criticizing medical care are actually contradictory. It is only the stagnation of mass movements in the present period that makes them seem incompatible: if there were a large-scale popular demand for improved health care, the two critiques would not appear to be in conflict. And conversely, it is only by connecting

the two critiques that such a popular movement is possible. Let us examine these assertions.

First, neither the demands growing out of the political economic critique nor the demands growing out of the cultural critique can be realized save through a mass movement. In the case of the political economic demands, this is perhaps self-evident: the vested power of the doctors, drug companies, insurance companies, etc. can only be overcome through a massive popular upsurge. On the face of the matter, some of the demands growing out of the cultural critique—e.g., for a health system based on more self-help, for less dependency on professional medical care, for an approach to health emphasizing the importance of personal habits such as eating, exercise, smoking, etc.—do not appear to require such confrontations with economic and political power. But they do require major changes in how people perceive themselves, their bodies, their relationships to others; they do require the unleashing of people's imaginations. And it is only under conditions of massive involvement in a social movement that these changes are likely to occur.

Moreover, a mass popular movement could readily embrace the demands growing out of both critiques. The sixties provide a relevant model: as we have seen, the cultural critique grew in large measure out of the radical community and feminist movements of this period. This suggests that the notion advanced above, that the political economic demand for "more" grows out of scarcity and that the cultural demand for "different" grows out of plenty is, perhaps, too simple and static. Mounting scarcity can beget passivity, as we have seen repeatedly in the last few years. And it is the perception that "more" is *possible*, even though it has not yet been *achieved*, that stimulates people to examine their own experience, to imagine how they would like services to be, and hence to experiment with alternatives (e.g., alternate institutions, insurgent operation of existing institutions). In the absence of a mass movement to demand better health care, then, the demands stemming from the two modes of criticism of medical care seem opposed. But the opposition is illusory: it disappears in the context of a popular movement.

Finally, it seems to me hard to imagine that any large and

effective movement could develop if it did not emphasize *both* the need for more services *and* the need for a different approach to health altogether. A movement cannot develop if it does not offer people the hope of meeting perceived needs which now go unmet. But if people also perceive that there is something very wrong with even the services that they have, they will not be drawn into a movement that only offers them more of the same. The lack of mass enthusiasm (though not of vague, passive support) for national health insurance is instructive: why should anyone get excited about another bureaucracy to help them pay for services which they know are inadequate? Conversely, would not a movement which held out the vision not of more hospital beds and clinics but of a caring society, not of paying for ever more medical care but of reducing dependency on medical institutions, be infinitely more likely to capture people's imaginations?

Now, imagining the possibility of such a movement, we are led to ask in more detail what the nature of a socialist health system would be. Going back to the political economic and cultural critiques, it is evident that a socialist health system would offer high quality, dignified, readily available health services of all kinds on an equitable basis, regardless of geographic location, race, nationality, or ability to pay. (Although it is beyond my scope here to argue the case fully, if such a system is not to become a bottomless pit for money and to place its institutional priorities ahead of its patients' needs, it must take the form of a decentralized, community- and worker-controlled national health service rather than either national health insurance or a uniform, bureaucratically centralized national health service.) It is equally evident that we cannot talk about a socialist health system that does not deal with the social and environmental causes of bad health. At a minimum (!) this means eliminating poverty, poor housing, poor nutrition, poor schools; eliminating or sharply reducing air and water pollution; and combating unhealthy life styles (e.g., smoking, lack of exercise).

But this does not exhaust our notion of what a socialist (as opposed to a merely socialized) health system would look like. To inquire further, we must peel away the mystification of medical

care imposed by its complex technology and by its historical appearance as a commodity. Medical care is fundamentally a social, not a technical or commercial, relationship. It is embedded in the social relationships of the overall society and expresses the values of the broader society. To ask what kind of medical care we want is, then, to ask some very basic questions about the kind of society that we want to live in. We are left, as we suggested at the beginning of this essay, with the fundamental *social* question of how a good society deals with human *biological* interdependency: with death, birth, pain; with care of the young, the sick, the disabled, and the aged. I should like to conclude this essay by exploring a few of the questions about medical care that such a perspective suggests.

The problem of dependency. The cultural critique focused attention on the way in which the medical system fosters and abuses dependency. To take an extreme case, Ivan Illich has argued that increasing access to medical care would merely increase what he considers socially debilitating individual dependency, and has called for a radical demedicalizing of society; people should learn to cope autonomously with pain, sickness, disability. Illich's demand finds echo in the growing demand by many people for autonomous control over their own bodies, even in situations that doctors would consider deserving of major medical intervention: the number of home deliveries is rising rapidly; the self-help concept spreads; and a variety of health "fads" (e.g., for herbal remedies and massage therapies) have reached epidemic proportions. But, as I have argued above, some, at least, of medical technology is useful and inappropriate for use by untrained people. Rejecting this is, at the very least, a self-destructive form of "autonomy." In any case, the replacement of dependency on doctors with dependency on midwives, friends, and so forth is not a rejection of dependency *per se*; it is a *redirecting* of dependency.

How can the needs for autonomy and dependency be reconciled? The major problem of the medical system now is not that it generates dependency; the problem is the kind of dependency that it generates, and its social impact. What we have to develop is a medical system which acknowledges our need for autono-

mous control over our bodies *and* which accepts our need for dependency; which enhances autonomy but, when we do feel the necessity to give up and be dependent, can deal with that need in a dignified and nurturing way.

More broadly, we might ask whether the medical system should be the major mechanism for dealing with biological dependency. In the last half century or so, the medical system has increasingly assumed this role, taking over from the disintegrating family and community. Any society needs institutions to deal with dependency: the existence of mutual dependency with regard to biological functions is virtually the defining characteristic of human beings as social animals. It is natural, not morbid, that people sometimes need to be taken care of. But is the medical system the right institution to do this? If not, what alternatives are there? Do we imagine that the family, with appropriate social supporting mechanisms, can once again take over the care of the aged, the disabled? How useful, in this context, are images of the family drawn from other times (e.g., the patriarchal extended family of pre-industrial Europe) or from other places (e.g., the contemporary Chinese family, embedded in small, stable communities)? In any case, do we want to concentrate healing and caring in one institution, or spread it out throughout a variety of social institutions?

The problem of professionalism. In order to evolve a health system that is both a curing system and a caring system, we have to confront the problem of professionalism. In our system, professionalism is primarily a defense of status and privilege. Although doctors and other health professionals have defended professionalism as a bulwark of quality, it has functioned more effectively as a mechanism to protect the professionals from scrutiny, to limit access to the occupation and to medical knowledge, and to preserve doctors' control over the health system. To change the health system at all, much less to create a medical system which maximally utilizes self-help and mutual help and which encourages an active rather than a passive role for the patient, will require radical deprofessionalization. We will have to expand radically the use of community health aides; to spread medical knowledge to patients and to nonphysician health workers; to

minimize the social distance between doctors and patients. (I should emphasize that deprofessionalization has nothing to do with eliminating the *skills* of the doctors. Skills are of course needed, and I am not proposing that incompetent people perform medical services—we have too much of that as it is! It is the privileges, the power, and the monopolization of medical knowledge that I am speaking of removing when I speak of deprofessionalization.)

In another sense, however, we have to *re*professionalize medical care. Another of the traditional components of professionalism is the idea that providing health care is a calling, attended by a strong ethic of service. But the result of years of control of the medical system by the doctors in their own narrow self-interest has been the spread of widespread apathy, cynicism, even callousness among nonphysician health workers, who have seen the impossibility of delivering decent health care under our present health system. It seems to me urgent to build a health system in which the idea of health care as a *calling* can be restored. In the context of a capitalist society, however, the idea of selfless caring is considered masochistic. Stating this reemphasizes the magnitude of the social transformation required to have a humane health system: if socialized medicine means health care delivered by callous bureaucracies such as that of so many of our public hospitals and clinics today, we can hardly wonder that it fails to arouse public enthusiasm.

The problem of technology. What part of the technology of modern medicine is salvageable? Recall that a significant proportion of medicine's proudest claims to effectiveness may be false, and that a not insignificant part of modern medical practice may, on net, do more physical harm than good. In any case, in actual practice, much of what doctors do is not based on scientifically validated knowledge. (For instance, a National Academy of Sciences panel, studying the evidence for effectiveness of prescription drugs marketed in the United States in the mid-sixties, found that fully one half of these drugs were either ineffective or ineffective in the form normally prescribed, or at best, "possibly effective.") Doctors, despite their claims to be men of science, widely disregard scientific evidence. (For example, doctors go on

prescribing a drug such as the antibiotic Chloramphenicol in situations where its use is not indicated, despite the availability of alternative drugs and despite the widely publicized and occasionally lethal side effects of the drug.) And doctors, with rare exceptions, have been completely unable to recognize, much less deal with, the interactions of mind and body, environment and body, society and body.

The question, then, is not one of throwing out scientific medicine; it is a question of whether medicine can *become* a science. This, in turn, raises questions about the basic assumptions of science (in the sense of physics, chemistry, biology): the traditional natural sciences objectify the things that they study; they have no place for consciousness or subjectivity. But human beings are conscious creatures; as I have repeatedly emphasized, the healing relationship is not merely physiological, but also social. Are biology and chemistry and physics an adequate, appropriate, and complete basis for a science of healing human beings? If not, what is the basis (or what are the limitations) of scientific medicine? The conditions of medical practice in capitalist society have not permitted this question to be raised seriously.

Medicine as a social endeavor. In repudiating our present dependency on institutionalized medicine for all aspects of health care, it would be easy to embrace the opposite extreme—medical anarchy: notions of rationality in determining methods of care, of discipline in obtaining and using skills, of belief in medical authority would be discarded; what feels good, physically or psychologically, would become the arbiter of the kind of medical care that one would seek. Already signs of such a revolt against medicine as a rational and social endeavor abound, evidenced for example in the booming demand for almost certainly useless drugs such as Laetrile, and in the widespread reliance on home remedies for serious and readily treatable ailments. (The irony is great: the same people who berate the drug companies for their lack of testing or their false advertising of drugs embrace and extol the value of totally untested herbal remedies.)*

---

* In China, where efforts to inculcate rationalist, scientific modes of thinking in people are a high priority, a high-ranking health official told me that he regarded

How, then, do we reconcile notions of individual freedom and dignity with a rational and social approach to healing technology? Should people have the right to do whatever they want to their bodies? (For example, should the prescription system be abolished and all drugs be freely available over the counter?) Should practitioners have the right to treat illnesses in whatever manner they deem appropriate, and should patients have the right to choose anyone claiming to be a practitioner to treat them? If not, who should determine who is a competent healer and who is not? Other healers? Patients? Using what criteria?

Questions such as these make it clear that the problems of health and medicine cannot be treated as problems of technique, of administration, of distribution, separate from the overall problems of social values and the institutional arrangements by which the dominant classes in a society express their values. Even a brief effort at trying to define a socialist medicine reveals that questions of health policy are not narrow questions of how to reform the health system; they are among the most profound questions that we can ask about the society in which we live.

The essays in Part 1 explore the social functions of medicine from a theoretical point of view. Barbara and John Ehrenreich focus on the nature and consequences of the interaction between an individual doctor and his or her patients. Irving Zola examines why medicine has replaced institutions such as the family and the church as a mechanism of social control and discusses the political consequences of the "medicalization" of social problems. Marc Renaud locates some of the limitations of modern medicine in the models of human health and disease evolved by capitalist societies since the late nineteenth century.

Parts 2 and 3 are more empirical, providing together two case studies in the themes developed theoretically in Part 1. In Part 2 (Medicine and Women), Barbara Ehrenreich and Deirdre English sketch historically the role of doctors in controlling women's lives. Linda Gordon traces how one particular part of the technology associated with the control of women's lives—birth

---

double blind procedures for testing drugs and controlled studies of the relative effectiveness and the side effects of drugs for the same illness as "bourgeois" notions, reflecting drug companies' competitive interests. I was not convinced.

control—began to be taken out of women's hands and placed under physicians' control. Doris Haire argues that current medical approaches to childbirth in the United States have little basis in science; they are culturally, rather than technically, determined procedures. Mary Howell and Diana Scully and Pauline Bart suggest that doctors' sexist attitudes toward women pervade the medical literature and are inculcated in young doctors by their textbooks (among other means), with no regard for their scientific validity.

In Part 3 (Medicine and Imperialism), Frantz Fanon provides a classic description of how the overall social relations between an oppressor and an oppressed group pervade the medical interaction between doctors (belonging to the oppressor group) and patients (belonging to the oppressed group). Fanon's example is colonial Algeria, but his comments would apply equally well to blacks in the United States, to women, and to other oppressed groups. James Paul and E. Richard Brown discuss the historical uses of medicine in advancing U.S. and European imperialism. And Howard Levy describes the direct role that medicine came to play in the U.S. effort to suppress the revolutionary struggle in Vietnam. (Dr. Levy, many readers may recall, was jailed for two years for his refusal to teach Green Berets medical tricks to help "pacify" the Vietnamese.)

NOTES

1. See, for example, Committee on the Costs of Medical Care, *Medical Care for the American People* (Chicago: University of Chicago Press, 1932; reprinted by the U.S. Dept. of Health, Education, and Welfare, Washington, D.C., 1970). More recent examples include Edward M. Kennedy, *In Critical Condition* (New York: Simon & Schuster, 1972); Abraham Ribicoff with P. Danaceau, *The American Medical Machine* (New York: Saturday Review Press, 1972); Ed Cray, *In Failing Health* (Indianapolis and New York: Bobbs-Merrill, 1970).

2. See Barbara and John Ehrenreich, *The American Health Empire: Power, Profits, and Politics* (A Health-PAC book; New York: Random House, 1970); *Billions for Bandaids*, ed. T. Bodenheimer, S. Cummings, and E. Harding (San Francisco: Medical Committee for Human Rights, 1972); *Prognosis Negative: Crisis in the Health Care*

System, ed. David Kotelchuck (A Health-PAC book; New York: Vintage, 1976); Vicente Navarro, *Medicine Under Capitalism* (New York: Prodist, 1976). Navarro argues that it is not private ownership per se but the institutional and ideological subordination of the health sector to the ruling classes of American capitalism which determine the characteristics of American medicine.

3. See Henry E. Sigerist, "Socialized Medicine," *The Yale Review* (Spring 1938), reprinted in *National Health Care*, ed. Ray H. Elling (New York: Lieber-Atherton, 1973); Milton Roemer, "Nationalized Medicine for America," *Trans-Action* (September 1971); Medical Committee for Human Rights, "Preliminary Position Paper on National Health Care" (September 1971), reprinted by Congressman Ron V. Dellums in *Congressional Record*, vol. 117, no. 199, part III, December 17, 1971.

4. H. J. Eysenck, "Effects of Psychotherapy," *International Journal of Psychiatry* 1 (1965): 97-198; also, Philip R. A. May, *Treatment of Schizophrenia* (New York: Science House, 1968), esp. pp. 47-52; and L. Grinspoon, J. R. Ewalt, and R. Shader, "Psychotherapy and Pharmacotherapy in Chronic Schizophrenia," *American Journal of Psychiatry* 124 (1968): 1645-52.

5. R. D. Laing, "The Obvious," in *Going Crazy*, ed. Hendrik M. Ruitenbeck (New York: Bantam Books, 1972), p. 113.

6. Thomas Szasz, *The Myth of Mental Illness*, rev. ed. (New York: Harper and Row, 1974), pp. 69 and 267. See also Thomas Szasz, *The Manufacture of Madness* (New York: Dell, 1970); R. D. Laing, *The Politics of Experience* (New York: Ballantine, 1967); R. D. Laing, *The Divided Self* (Baltimore: Penguin, 1965); Phyllis Chesler, *Women and Madness* (Garden City, N.Y.: Doubleday, 1972); E. Fuller Torrey, *The Death of Psychiatry* (Radnor, Pa.: Chilton, 1974); Naomi Weisstein, "Psychology Constructs the Female," in *Women in Sexist Society*, ed. V. Gornick and B. K. Moran (New York: Signet/New American Library, 1971).

7. Leslie A. Falk, "The Negro American's Health and the Medical Committee for Human Rights," *Medical Care* 4 (July-September 1966): 171-77; Pierre deVise et al., *Slum Medicine: Chicago's Apartheid Health System* (Chicago: Community and Family Study Center, University of Chicago, 1969); Roger Hurley, "The Health Crisis of the Poor," in *The Social Organization of Health*, ed. Hans Peter Dreitzel (New York: Macmillan, 1971); J. M. Gayles, Jr., "Health Brutality and the Black Life Cycle," *The Black Scholar* (May 1974): Bonnie Bullough and Vern L. Bullough, *Poverty, Ethnic Iden-*

tity, and Health Care (New York: Appleton-Century-Crofts, 1972); U.S. Dept. of Health, Education, and Welfare, *Bibliography of Racism*, DHEW Publication No. (ADM) 76-318, (Washington, D.C., 1976).

8. See Emily Spieler, "Division of Laborers," *Health-PAC Bulletin* (November 1972); C. A. Brown, "The Division of Laborers: Allied Health Professions," *International Journal of Health Services* 3, no.3 (1973); Barbara Ehrenreich and John Ehrenreich, "Hospital Workers: Class Conflicts in the Making," *International Journal of Health Services* 5, no. 1 (1975); John B. McKinlay, "On the Professional Regulation of Change," *Sociological Review Monograph No. 20*, University of Keele, Staffordshire, England (1973).

9. On the Topeka story, see Alex Efthim, "We Care in Kansas: The Non-Professionals Revolt," *The Nation*, August 5, 1968. On Lincoln Hospital, see Barbara and John Ehrenreich, *The American Health Empire*, chap. 18; and "Lincoln Hospital: Three Views," *Health Rights News* (January 1971). On free clinics, see Barbara and John Ehrenreich, *The American Health Empire*, chap. 17; Source Collective, *Organizing for Health Care* (Boston: Beacon, 1974), pp. 8-18; and "Free Clinics," *Health-PAC Bulletin* (October 1971).

10. In addition to the articles included in this volume, see Boston Women's Health Collective, *Our Bodies, Ourselves* New York: Simon & Schuster, 1972); Ellen Frankfurt, *Vaginal Politics* (New York: Quadrangle, 1972); Barbara Seaman, *Free and Female* (Garden City, N.Y.: Doubleday, 1972); Barbara Ehrenreich and Deirdre English, *Witches, Midwives, and Nurses: A History of Women Healers* (Old Westbury, N.Y.: The Feminist Press, 1973); Barbara Ehrenreich and Deidre English, *Complaints and Disorders: The Sexual Politics of Sickness* (Old Westbury, N.Y.: The Feminist Press, 1973). Bibliographies of recent writings on women and medicine can be found in Jane B. Sprague, "Women and Health Bookshelf," *American Journal of Public Health* 65 (July 1975): 741-46; and *Women and Health Care: A Bibliography with Selected Annotation*, Program on Women, Northwestern University, Evanston, Ill., 1975.

11. René Dubos, *The Mirage of Health* (New York: Harper and Row, 1959); René Dubos, *Man Adapting* (New Haven: Yale University Press, 1965); Thomas McKeown, *Medicine in Modern Society* (London: Allen and Unwin, 1965); John Powles, "On the Limitations of Modern Medicine," *Science, Medicine, and Man* 1 (1973); A. L. Cochrane, *Effectiveness and Efficiency: Random Reflections on Health Services* (London: Oxford, 1972).

12. René Dubos, *Man, Medicine, and Environment* (New York: Mentor, 1968); Hans Selye, *The Stress of Life*, rev. ed. (New York: McGraw-Hill, 1976); Leo W. Simmons and Harold G. Wolff, *Social Science in Medicine* (New York: Russell Sage Foundation, 1954). On the relative lack of interest of physicians in the social, psychological, and environmental aspects of medicine, see G. Gordon, O. W. Anderson, H. P. Brehm, and S. Marquis, *Disease: The Individual and Society* (New Haven: College and University Press, 1968).

13. Barbara Seaman, *The Doctor's Case Against the Pill* (New York: Peter H. Wyden, 1969).

14. Ivan Illich, *Medical Nemesis: The Expropriation of Health* (New York: Pantheon, 1976), pp. 3 and 26. Additional references to the literature on clinical iatrogenesis can be found in *Medical Nemesis*, pp. 13-36.

15. Ibid., p. 41.

16. Karl Marx and Friedrich Engels, *The German Ideology* (New York: International Publishers, 1947), pp. 16 and 18.

17. Joshua Horn, *Away With All Pests* (New York: Monthly Review Press, 1971); Victor Sidel and Ruth Sidel, *Serve the People* (Boston: Beacon Press, 1974).

18. Illich, *Medical Nemesis*, p. 74.

19. *Infant Death: An Analysis by Maternal Risk and Health Care* (Washington, D.C.: Institute of Medicine, National Academy of Science, 1973); also see Victor Fuchs, *Who Shall Live?* (New York: Basic Books, 1975), pp. 31-55.

20. See note 11.

21. See, for instance, M. I. Roemer and S. J. Axelrod, "A National Health Service and Social Security," *American Journal of Public Health* 67 (1977): 462-65.

22. See, for instance, Navarro, *Medicine Under Capitalism*, pp. 126-28.

PART 1

THE SOCIAL FUNCTIONS OF MEDICINE: SOME THEORETICAL CONSIDERATIONS

BARBARA AND JOHN EHRENREICH
MEDICINE AND SOCIAL CONTROL

The question most frequently addressed to angry groups of service consumers in the sixties was: "What do you people *really* want?" The initial answers could be condensed to one word: more—more educational opportunities, more health and mental health services, more welfare and social services. In time, the answers were tempered with the realization that "more" might be less than enough, and even "better" might not be good enough. What was the point of more schools, or even more teachers and equipment per school, if the fundamental mission of the schools was to socialize children into capitalist values and (unappealing) work roles? Who wants a community mental health center, even an attractive and well-staffed one, if its ultimate prescription for mental health is acquiescence to oppression? As a radical analysis developed and deepened, it made it clear that the schools, the welfare agencies, and the mental health and other social service systems were agencies of *social control*. "More" was not only not enough; it could be dangerous.

The one area of human services which escaped the sixties relatively unsmeared was medicine. It is true that radicals (ourselves included) bitterly castigated the medical system, but always more for what it did *not* do than for what it did. It did not offer high-quality, dignified medical care to the poor; it did not energetically expand preventive services; it did not lower the financial barriers to the care experienced by working-class people. Why not? The answer was simple enough: the medical system was too concerned with profits, power, and status to care much about services; these were merely a byproduct of Americas' "number

one growth industry"—health. Radical analysis tended to ignore the byproduct and focused on the industry—its institutional contours, its relationship to government and the economy in general, etc.[1]

If there was a "politics of health" that went deeper than the political economy of the institutions and the gross inequities in the availability of care, it was not examined. Medical services themselves were seen as politically neutral: the need for them was biologically ordained; their precise content was technologically determined. Although all the visible abuses—profiteering, unjust distribution, the use of poor people as "teaching material," racism and sexism from doctors, and so forth—came under fire, the core of the system remained sacrosanct, out of bounds for social criticism.

There are two important exceptions—two areas where radical analysis has gone beyond a single-minded concern with availability and quality and begun to probe the ideological content of health services themselves. First there is the area of mental health. Early critiques of mental health services focused on their unavailability to poor and working-class people. Today, many radical psychiatrists are skeptical about the therapeutic value of conventional mental health services for anyone. They have arrived at the conclusion that mental health services operate directly to enforce oppressive sex and class roles, to reinforce individualism, and to promote the idea that however oppressive your situation is, your problems are "all in your head."[2]

The second area in which the health movement has broached the issue of the ideology of health care is the area of women's medical care. Faced with what some have described as "sexocidal" tendencies in medicine—evidenced by massive pharmaceutical experiments on women, excessive gynecological surgery, and so forth—it is not surprising that the overwhelming concern of the women's health movement is *survival*. As in the health movement in general, availability, cost, and quality are the central issues. At the same time, the ideological content of the services has not gone unexamined. Feminists point out that the treatment of women is often patriarchal to the point of medical irrationality. (For example, standard obstetrical procedure features the woman unconscious and/or strapped down to a table

while the lordly obstetrician extracts the baby with forceps. There is considerable evidence that anesthesia, the supine position, and forceps are unhealthy for mother and baby.) The effect of this kind of treatment is to promote feelings of passivity and low self-worth on the part of women, hence to reinforce oppressed roles as wives and workers.[3]

But the issues raised by feminists and radical mental health workers have not been integrated into the mainstream of radical analysis of the medical system. They have been incorporated as qualifications, and little more: "We want *more*, but, if possible, without the sexism, racism, ideological manipulation, etc." Whether such a qualified expansion is possible, whether the ideologically objectionable features of the services can simply be "peeled off" the presumably neutral core, has not been examined. Answering such questions, it seems to us, is central to the framing of a truly socialist, feminist, and humanist vision of health care.

Our purpose here is to lay out a tentative approach to an understanding of the social control functions of the medical system. At the outset we want to make clear, first, that our approach is sociological, and not primarily medical or economic. We are not concerned with the biological impact of medical services, but with their social impact—how they are viewed by people, what expectations people bring to them, how their behavior or understanding of social reality is affected by them. Thus we would not ask of a given service, or element of service, such as a chest x-ray: "Was it really necessary or helpful?" It might well be both necessary and helpful, but regardless of the answer, we are interested in a different set of questions: how was it experienced by the patient? What was the nature of the social interactions required for its performance? Though some may see this approach as narrow or blind to everything that is "good" in medicine, we see it as essential to making a fresh start in our analysis—to seeing medicine as something other than what the medical men themselves define it as. And except insofar as the financial transactions between doctor (or hospital) and patient directly affect the social relations between them, we shall not be concerned with the economics of health care, either.

Second, our description of the medical system as a system of

social control is not, in itself, an attack on the medical system. *Any* social system is characterized by mechanisms of social control—mechanisms that ensure that members of the society follow the behavior patterns acceptable to the particular society (in particular, in the societies we are most familiar with, to the ruling classes of the society—but even a totally egalitarian society would have such mechanisms). Our concern here is not with the fact that the medical system functions as a system of social control *per se*; it is rather with the *content* of the social control exercised. To sum up our argument briefly, a capitalist health-care system operates to maintain and reinforce capitalist social relations.

Third, we should make it clear that to analyze something as a system of social control is not to view it as a conspiracy. We are not arguing that the health system is consciously designed to exercise social control, or that the social control functions of the health system somehow explain its structure and dynamics. On the contrary, we explain the social control functions as themselves a result of the institutional structure, organization, and economics of the health-care system.

Finally, we want to emphasize that our analysis is a tentative one, bordering in places on the purely speculative. The value of such a tentative beginning lies in the work which it stimulates others to do.

THE SOCIOLOGY OF MEDICINE

Doctors (and most of the public) view the medical system as a system for distributing technical expertise and intervention in the interest of improved biological fitness among the recipients. *Sociologists* view the medical system as a system of social relationships: "sickness" is a *social role* (as opposed to "disease," which is a *biological state*) and it is the business of the medical system to control entry into sick roles and to define the behavior appropriate to them. In the medical view, the issue of social control never arises, unless one considers that making people fit or capable to perform their normal activities is in itself a form of social "control." In the sociological view, the medical system is,

at least in a formal sense, a system of "social control"—simply because it defines roles, regulates entry into them, etc. Our interest here is not in academic formalisms—sociological or medical—but in the social and ideological impact of the medical system. We take some of the conclusions of academic sociology as a starting point for our analysis because they provide important insights into the fundamentally *political* issues that concern us: who is being "controlled," by whom, how, and in whose interests? And although such questions may not be of great concern to bourgeois sociology, we emphasize that they cannot even be framed within the *medical* description of the medical system which has so thoroughly dominated radical thinking up until now.

The two most important contributers to the sociological description of medicine are Talcott Parsons and Eliot Freidson.[4] We have no intention of summarizing, much less criticizing, their work, but we would like briefly to restate what we have found important in it. We consider them separately because their views, while in no way considered contradictory in sociological circles, do imply two apparently contradictory descriptions of the medical system and of the forms of social control that it exerts.

Parsons' classic contribution to medical sociology is his description of the sick role. The characteristics of the sick role are: (1) The individual is not held responsible for his/her condition. (Sinners and criminals are responsible; sick people are not.) (2) Conditions defined as illness are seen as a legitimate basis for certain *exemptions* from normal responsibilities—"sick" people can stay home from work, be waited on, etc., depending on the severity of the incapacity. (3) The exemptions held out to sick persons are only *conditionally* legitimate, the prime condition being that the sick person recognize that sickness is an undesirable state and that he/she has an obligation to try to get well. (4) In our society, this is an obligation to seek competent help and to cooperate completely with the efforts of competent helpers in becoming well.

In Parsons' view the sick role is always a tempting one: it is not considered blameworthy and it offers a way out of normal responsibilities. Insofar as illness is motivated, "the motives which enter into illness as deviant behavior are partially identical with those

entering into other types of deviance, such as crime and the breakdown of commitment to the values of society. . . ." So it is understandable that certain features of the social construction of sickness are set up to discourage people from using a sickness as a way of dropping out:

> Life has necessarily become more complex and has made greater demands on the typical individual. . . . The motivation to retreat into ill-health through mental or psychosomatic channels, has become accentuated and with it the importance of effective mechanisms for coping with those who do so retreat.

First, there is the fact that sickness is seen as undesirable:

> The stigmatizing of illness as undesirable and the mobilization of considerable resources of the community to combat illness is a reaffirmation of the valuation of health and a countervailing influence against the temptation for illness. . . . Thus the sick person is prevented from setting an example which others might be tempted to follow.

As an added precaution, the sick are insulated from each other and from the general public, and placed under the supervision of certain nonsick people (medical personnel):

> The essential reason for this insulation being important in the present context is not the need of the sick person for special "care" so much as it is that, motivationally as well as bacteriologically, illness may well be contagious.[5]

The picture of the American "sickness system" that emerges from Parsons' work, then, is like nothing so much as the American welfare system. Welfare too holds out exemptions, particularly from the requirement to seek gainful employment. But these exemptions are offered only to the "legitimately" poor (those certified as eligible) and they are only offered on the condition that the recipients recognize their state as undesirable and cooperate with "competent helpers" (social workers) to overcome the "character defects," "family pathology," etc., which have led to it. Like the sick role, the "welfare role" puts the recipient under the supervision of certain nonpoor people (caseworkers). And, even more obviously than in the case of sickness, a variety of

measures (low payments, degrading procedures) are taken to make sure that the welfare role will not be too tempting to the mass of working people. Concern for the sick or poor, it seems, must always be held in check by the fearful possibility of *contagion*.[6]

Singularly absent from Parsons' description is any sense of agency. What determines the "social construction of sickness" that he describes? In the homogeneous and seemingly middle-class America of Parsons' medical writings, the answer is simply "our values," and these appear to arise out of some deep cultural consensus. The first thing that strikes us as important about Freidson's work is that he identifies the actual architects of our "social construction of sickness": it is the medical profession that defines illness in theory (i.e., defines which biological syndromes admit one to the sick roles and which can be considered as minor, psychosomatic, or otherwise ineligible for special treatment). And it is the doctors who identify illness in practice (determine who is eligible for sick roles), and undertake to supervise those identified as "sick."

> They [professionals] are not merely experts but incumbents in official positions. . . . Given the official status of the profession, what happens to the layman—that is, whether or not he will be recognized as "really" sick, what the sickness will be called, what treatment will be given him, how he will be required to act while ill, and what will happen to him after treatment—becomes a function of professional rather than lay decision. . . . Thus the behavior of the physician and others in the field of health constitutes the objectification, the empirical embodiment, of certain dominant values in a society.[7]

Where Parsons is concerned with a culturally diffuse "sickness system" (our term), Freidson is concerned with the actual medical system. He describes it as an agency of social control on a par with the legal system or organized religion. Each of these institutions is concerned with the prevention, detection, and management of social deviance—criminality in the case of the law, sin in the case of the church, sickness in the case of the medical system. In his understanding of deviance, Freidson makes a significant

departure from Parsons. Parsons sees deviance as motivated behavior or deliberate idiosyncrasy—more a matter for psychiatry than for sociology to comprehend. Freidson's approach is operational; he describes deviance as a state *imputed* by the relevant officials: the courts label certain people as "murderers" or "shoplifters"; doctors label certain others as "cancer cases" or "neurotics." Once so labeled, the person is required to enter the social role appropriate to the label—to undergo certain types of treatment, to modify his or her behavior in ways seen as therapeutic, perhaps to abandon all other social roles and enter an institution filled with similarly labeled people (cancer ward, jail, mental hospital).

The aspect of the sick role which seemed to concern Parsons was the exemptions that it entailed, and the allure that these might exercise on the nonsick. The aspect of the sick role that concerns Freidson is the requirement that the sick person cooperate with the agencies and personnel set up to deal with his or her sickness. To enter the sick role is to enter a state of professional dominance:

> In essence, the process of treatment and care may be seen as a process which attempts to lead the patient to behave in the way considered appropriate to the illness which has been diagnosed, a process often called "management" by professionals. . . . Professional management generally functions *to remove from the patient his identity as an adult, self-determining person*, and to press him to serve the moral and social identity implied by the illness which is diagnosed. [Emphasis added][8]

This is a remarkably cold-blooded description of the sick role, and one that raises serious political—if not moral—issues.

What does arouse Freidson's moral concern is not the power of the medical profession to manage the sick, but its power to define what is "sick." He describes the medical system as continually expanding its definition of sickness to embrace more and more forms of social deviance: sin is going out of style along with the church; the courts are losing ground to the psychiatric establishment; and "the hospital is succeeding the church and the parliament as the archetypical institution of Western culture."[9] Drunkenness becomes "alcoholism"; "perversion" becomes "psy-

chosis"; and so on as medicine expands its jurisdiction to cover more and more areas once reserved for law or religion:

> The consequence of the movement [expansion of medicine's jurisdiction], however, is the strengthening of a professionalized control institution that, in the name of the individual's good and of technical expertise, can remove from laymen the right to evaluate their own behavior and the behavior of their fellow—a fundamental right that is evidenced in a hard-won fight to interpret the Scriptures oneself, without regard to dogmatic authority, in religion and, the right to be judged by one's peers, in law.[10]

The picture of the medical system that emerges from Freidson's description is that of some vast, expansionist, and itself uncontrolled regulatory apparatus—forever advancing the frontiers of its jurisdiction and enfolding more and more citizens into its (always benevolent) supervision. Medical theory aggressively claims new territory as "sickness." Practicing physicians zealously recruit their patients into sick roles (lest they miss someone who turns out to be "really sick" after all). The ranks of the "sick" swell, but there is no way that this army of "deviants" can turn against the social order; each marches to a separate drummer, and submits to his or her own medical "management."

There is a world of difference between this and Parsons' vision of the medical system (or, to be fair, our extrapolation of his vision). The one is chary in its favors (exemptions); the other is recklessly indulgent. The one excites moral concern over what it may not do, whom it may not care for, in its caution lest "sickness" sap the moral fiber of the nation. The other excites concern for what it *does* do, whom it does care for, in its drive to be caretaker for more and more of the nation's ills.

We emphasize this difference in perspective not because we are interested in provoking an academic sociological debate where there was none before, but because the same apparent contradiction runs through the radical critiques of the medical system: on the one hand we blame the system for being too chary and exclusionary—"there are not enough services; what there are are too costly, uninviting," etc." On the other hand we, to a lesser extent, blame the system for being expansionist—claiming ever

more areas for its jurisdiction and endlessly expanding its institutional apparatus. Nowhere is this contradiction closer to the surface than in the critiques of "medical empires."[11] Some empires were criticized for being "conservative" and failing to expand their services to needy communities. Others were criticized for being "expansionist" and seeking to expand their services—i.e., their "control" over community health resources. Some were criticized for having *both* tendencies.

We do not wish to make too much of this apparent inconsistency. As activists learned in the health movement, the medical system does have both exclusionary and expansionist faces, and neither is wholly benign, or even "neutral." In fact, we can now postulate that the expansionist and exclusionary aspects of the medical system, recognized by both academic sociologists and radical critics, correspond to two different forms of *social control* exerted by the medical system, which we shall call *disciplinary* social control and *cooptative* social control.

TYPES OF MEDICAL SOCIAL CONTROL

Disciplinary control.   This type of social control is exerted by exclusionary sectors of the medical system. Exclusionary sectors are characterized by high barriers to entry (high costs, geographical inaccessibility, etc.) or socially repellent treatment of those who do enter (discourtesy, extreme impersonality, racism, fragmentation of care, long waits, etc.). The impact of exclusionary sectors on the populations that they are supposed to serve is to discourage entry into sick roles, either because of the visible barriers to entry or because of public knowledge of the treatment experienced by those who do enter (or, in some cases, both). In so doing, such services exert what we will call disciplinary social control in that they *encourage* people to maintain work or family responsibilities—no matter what subjective discomfort they may be experiencing.

Disciplinary social control operates primarily on those who are not "sick" (in the sociological, not the medical sense). At times, it has been used quite consciously to maintain industrial discipline in the work force. Foucault describes the combined poorhouses/

insane asylums of eighteenth- and nineteenth-century Paris and London. These were maintained as *public spectacles* to remind the populace of what awaited them if they opted to drop out into pauperism or madness. [12] In much the same way today, exposés of conditions in state mental hospitals serve to discourage "madness" as an out, just as public knowledge of the indignities inflicted on welfare recipients serves to discourage willful unemployment. (Doctors also may function quite explicitly to keep people out of sick roles and in work roles rather than to detect and cure disease. Consider the company doctor, whose role is to pressure the injured worker to return to his station: production losses are minimized and the company saves on workman's compensation benefits. The widespread requirement of a "doctor's note" to excuse absence from work or school similarly reflects the anti-"malingering" function of the medical system.)

Cooptative control. This kind of social control is exerted by expansionary sectors of the medical system. Expansionary sectors are characterized by relatively low barriers to entry, and acceptable, even sympathetic, treatment of those who do enter. Such services encourage people both to enter sick roles and to seek professional help in a variety of nonsick situations (for preventive care, contraceptive services, marital difficulties, etc.). In so doing they bring large numbers of people into the fold of *professional management* of various aspects of their lives. It is this situation of professional management—whether all-inclusive, as in the case of a cancer patient, or partial—which allows for the exercise of cooptative control. It should be clear that cooptative control, unlike disciplinary control, operates on those who do gain entry into the system, to whatever degree. The important question, of course, is: What is the nature and ideological content of cooptative control? In other words, what is the impact of professional management on the patient's ideology, self-image, acceptance of work and family roles, etc.? We will devote a major section of this paper to a discussion of these questions.

First, however, it is important to emphasize that the exclusionary and expansionist aspects of the medical system are often closely intermingled. A given agency, or even physician, may present exclusionary or expansionist faces at different times, in

different situations, to different groups of patients. At the same time, as we all know, there are certain consistent patterns in the kind of care experienced by different groups in our society— classes, sexes, races, age groups. For example, the overwhelming historical experience of the poor is of an exclusionary system. Thus the different forms of social control that we have distinguished are exerted differentially on different groups in society. History provides a striking illustration of the differential social control functions of the medical system.

Consider the kinds of medical care experienced by the urban poor and by the urban upper and upper-middle classes in late nineteenth-century America. (This period is interesting not only because it provides such vivid contrasts but because this is the period of the formation of the American medical profession.) The urban poor—mostly first- and second-generation immigrant workers—faced a grossly exclusionary system. Aside from a few dispensaries located in the ghettos, professional out-patient care was virtually unavailable; doctors were not interested in serving people who could not pay, or could not pay well. Institutional care, in the few municipal hospitals of the time, was avoided for good reasons—sanitary conditions in the hospitals were atrocious; nursing care was minimal until quite late in the century; and medical science had little to offer anyway.

Professionally "legitimized" sick roles were simply not available to the poor. Grinding poverty and the brutality of employers meant that if you were sick enough not to work, you were probably sick enough to die, and conditions in the hospitals meant that if you were going to die, you were better off dying at home. *Disease*, of course, *was* readily available to the poor—TB, cholera, typhus and typhoid fevers, malnutrition, and untreated complications of childbirth were rampant. But without a social and medical system willing to identify the diseased and offer exemptions to them, disease does not become sickness—the diseased go right on working. Thus, to the extent that the nascent medical system of the time had any effect on the poor, it was to enforce industrial discipline.

Meanwhile, the urban upper classes—families of wealthy businessmen, bankers, etc.—faced a medical "system" that was ex-

pansionary to a degree experienced by very few Americans today. Relative to today, there was an *excess* of doctors serving the better-off. (At least it appeared so to the American Medical Association at a time when doctors were reduced to running newspaper ads and other less-than-professional tactics to drum up business.) One of the medical profession's most successful business strategies was the exploitation of affluent women as patients. First, medical theory maintained that women—or at least "ladies"—were inherently sick; menstruation (with or without any irregularity), pregnancy, menopause, and puberty were described as morbid conditions requiring close medical management. To fill in the time between these reproductive crises, doctors found a host of vague disorders—"nerves," "chlorosis," "hysteria"—also requiring diligent treatment. (Medical neglect of poor women, who also suffered from the supposedly baneful effect of uterus and ovaries, was justified on the grounds that the poor were constitutionally tougher than the rich, consistent with their "coarser" natures.)

Sickness became so stylish among upper-class women that it is hard to say where the sick role ended and the approved social role of women began. Fainting and nervous delicacy were signs of good breeding; lengthy rest cures and visits to health spas were definitely "in"; invalidism was virtually a way of life for many; the doctor was an almost constant companion. The woman who yearned for a more active life ran into stern medical admonishments—higher education could cause the uterus to atrophy; political involvement, even voting, could be an invitation to hysteria. Rebelliousness was itself pathological, and indicated the need for a medically managed return to "normalcy."

Whether the doctors were motivated by greed, misogyny, or a benevolent concern for the "weaker sex" does not concern us here. There can be no question but that medicine operated as a key agency in the social control of women—enforcing passivity and a childlike dependency on men, particularly on doctors and on the husbands who paid the bills. It is true that these women were *objectively* dependent on men anyway; they had few rights and no means of self-support. But medical theory provided a "scientific" justification for their dependency; and medical prac-

tice served, in effect, as an intimate surveillance system—ready to detect female discontent when it was still at the stage of "nerves" or hysteria, and to intervene at once with a regime for "recovery."[13]

Thus the emerging medical system exerted two different kinds of social control on the two groups that we have considered: services for the poor served as a warning to the poor not to get "sick" (and possibly to the rich, as a warning not to get poor). This is what we have termed "disciplinary" control, and was aimed at the not yet sick, the working poor. The wealthy, especially wealthy women, on the other hand, experienced what we term "cooptative" control. This form of control was latent in the services themselves, and directed at those labeled "sick" (a category which, in medical theory of the time, included all affluent women).

THE EVOLUTION OF THE MEDICAL SYSTEM

The differential pattern of social control which prevailed in the late nineteenth century cannot, of course, be simply extrapolated to the present. The class structure of society has changed dramatically; sex roles have changed in all social classes. Even more important, for our analysis, the medical system itself has undergone profound changes—not only since 1900, but since 1930. Two broad changes in the medical system seem particularly relevant: (1) the vast expansion of the system, in all dimensions; and (2) the rapid rise in status and class position of the medical profession. The first is related to an expansion of the cooptative social control exerted by the medical system; the second is related to changes in the ideological content of that control.

The expansion of the medical system since 1900, or even more strikingly, since 1930, needs little documentation. It can be measured with any parameter that one wishes to apply—the absolute and relative amount of money spent on medical services, the number of people employed by the medical system, the amount of institutional resources devoted to medicine, or the public utilization of medical services.[14] Underneath what appears to be an amorphous mushrooming, we can distinguish three major dimensions of expansion:

1. An expansion in the *jurisdiction* of the medical system to include totally new types of services and functions, and services which were not formerly seen as "medical": family planning, abortions, in-patient obstetrical care, long-term care of the aged and disabled, community mental health services, marriage and sex counseling, cosmetic surgery, etc.

2. An expansion in the *number and kinds of services* available within the traditional jurisdiction of medicine, along with a marked increase in the efficacy of these services. Thanks to biomedical technology, the medical system at last has "something to offer." Very little is left to "nature's course" any more, or considered hopeless. There are antibiotics for infections, radiation and chemotherapy for cancer, antihistamines for allergies, psychic energizers for depression, and surgery for just about anything.

3. An expansion in the *availability* of medical care along class lines. Medical care, though certainly not yet a right, is far from being a luxury. Medicaid, Blue Cross, and a host of other programs have put medical care within the financial reach of large numbers of poor and working-class people who would formerly have stood completely outside the medical system.

We will not attempt to analyze all of the social implications of medicine's expansion in these three dimensions. But one thing seems clear: the expansion of the medical system has been accompanied by a deepening public *dependency* on that system, and this dependency now extends, in varying degrees, to all strata of society. In the first place, the development of medical technology has produced a fantastic rise in public expectations of what the medical system has to offer.[15] Medical "miracles"—from heart transplants to kidney dialysis—promote the idea that almost any problem can be "cured." Headache? Take it to the doctor or take the pill that "doctors recommend." Recurrent cough? Maybe be cancer, but don't delay, the doctor has a cure. There is nothing too trivial to take to the doctor, and nothing too serious to be cured. At least to the middle class, death itself becomes almost an accident—a failure of technique.

Second, advances in medical technology have helped to pave the way for the *jurisdictional* expansion of the medical system, and this in turn has led to a great broadening and diffusion of the

public dependency on medicine. If medicine can "cure" anything from polio to TB, then why not dad's drinking problem, or mother's crankiness? The medical system is inexorably replacing lay sources of help (extended family members, neighbors, ministers) for problems ranging from how to handle a baby's cold to how to handle marital tensions or the burden of aged relatives. Even "Dear Abby," that steadfast holdout of lay wisdom, counsels all the really difficult cases to "see your family doctor." In part, this broadening dependency on medicine reflects real increases in the ability of medicine to deal with certain problems; in part it reflects basic changes in the pattern of American life: the breakdown of close-knit communities (especially for the recently suburbanized working class) and of extended families. The housewife isolated in an impersonal suburb may not *have* anyone to turn to except the doctor. But it is also true that doctors themselves encourage dependency by actively seeking to discredit lay advice and help—from chiropractic to "old wives' tales."

Health care is not, of course, the only human-service sector to expand in the last three decades; the educational system and the social welfare systems have grown apace. But the various service sectors differ markedly in the impact that rapid growth has had on their professional workers. The numbers of teachers and social workers have expanded as rapidly as have the services themselves. Along with rapid growth in numbers has gone a substantial measure of what has been called "proletarianization": teachers' and social workers' work has become more routinized, and the teachers and social workers themselves have become subject to closer and closer scrutiny by superiors. As a corollary of being treated more and more like "workers" and less and less like "professionals," both groups have rapidly accepted organization into unions in the last decade, and have conducted numerous widely reported strikes.

The case of the doctors is altogether different. The unique political power, tight organization, and traditional autonomy of doctors has enabled them to provide a greatly increased volume of services without significant increase in their own numbers. The doctor in solo practice has, as is well known, become a smaller and smaller component of the overall delivery of med-

icine; medical care delivery has increasingly shifted to institutions—the hospital, the clinic, the group practice, the community health center, and so forth. Within these institutional medical settings, the doctors represent a smaller and smaller proportion of all health workers. More and more of the tasks that traditionally would have been considered the doctors' are assigned instead to nurses, technicians, and administrators. But despite these changes, the doctors' power over the medical system remains virtually absolute. They have enormous administrative power within the institutional settings in which they practice. More important to our analysis, they remain the chief technical functionaries in the actual practice and public representations of medicine. It is still the medical profession which defines and identifies new diseases, diagnoses illness in individuals, and presides over the medical management of patients.

What is especially significant, the doctors have held on to their monopoly over communication with patients: nurses, technicians, and others may chat, but they cannot comment on your x-rays, or reveal so much as your temperature. In the eyes of the patient, the contributions of all other workers are secondary—only the doctor has the power to cure, or to pronounce you incurable.

By holding down their numbers and holding on to their power within an expanding system, the doctors have greatly improved their own incomes and standing in the American class structure. Back at the turn of the century, it was widely considered (by the doctors at least) that there was an excess of doctors. In rural areas and middle-class urban areas, doctors were certainly plentiful by today's standards. They often had good incomes, but few were wealthy men or men from wealthy backgrounds. Access to a career in medicine was relatively free compared to the present. As late as 1910, there were eight black medical schools and a substantial number of schools catering to women. Scores of "diploma mills" offered the title "doctor," if not serious medical training, to all comers at moderate cost.

In the first two decades of this century, however, opportunities for nonwealthy and nonwhite medical students almost vanished. The AMA and a few large foundations (notably the Carnegie

Foundation, which funded the famous Flexner Report on medical education, and the Rockefeller Foundation, which helped to implement the recommendations of the Flexner Report) waged a successful campaign to eliminate the greater number of the nation's medical schools, in the name of quality medical education. The results of this campaign were: (1) most of the schools catering to students other than upper-class white males were closed. This included all but two of the black medical schools and all but one of the women's schools. (Flexner, in his report, bewailed the fact that any "crude boy or jaded clerk" had been able to seek medical training.) (2) The cost of medical education sharply increased as medical schools installed laboratories, new equipment, etc. Again, poorer students were excluded. (3) A high school and college education became a prerequisite for medical training, again filtering out many prospective bright but poorer (or female or black) students. (4) The actual number of medical schools dropped rapidly from 162 in 1906 to 95 in 1916 and 79 in 1924; a drop in the number of doctors practicing in the communities soon followed. In 1900 there were 173 doctors for every 100,000 Americans. By 1920, there were only 137 and by 1930 only 125. [16]

From that time on until the late sixties, doctors were recruited primarily from upper- and upper-middle-class families. In 1967, for instance, 66 to 81 percent (depending on the category of medical school—public, private, etc.) of all medical students had fathers who were doctors, other professionals, or businessmen. As for practicing doctors, today 93 percent are men and more than 98 percent are white. [17]

And from the 1920s through the mid-sixties, the AMA kept a tight lid on the nation's supply of doctors by what the *Journal of the AMA*'s editors referred to as "professional birth control"— strict limiting of the number of medical school places. (We again emphasize that we are not concerned here with the technical impact of the reforms in medical education—i.e., whether or not they improved the quality of medical care, etc. We are concerned only with the sociological impact, which was to limit the number of doctors and to limit the sources of recruitment of doctors.)

The doctors did not reap the full benefits of their declining numbers until after the Depression was out of the way. Then,

with doctor supply limited and demand for health care soaring, their incomes rose dramatically, and with their incomes, their social standing. Consider: in the late 1920s and 1930s, doctors' average incomes were about on a par with those of dentists and lawyers; they were slightly over twice the average family incomes of the period and two-thirds higher than those of college teachers. By the 1960s, they had far outdistanced the lawyers and dentists. Their median incomes ($41,500 in 1970) were more than four times those of the average family and three-and-a-half times those of college teachers. A study in 1967 showed that the median assets of doctors aged in their fifties was $134,400. By comparison, the median assets for families with the head of the family aged 45 to 54 was $10,847. [18]

Data on doctors' social standing is more fragmentary, but suggestive. Recent studies of occupational prestige have shown doctors at the very top, on a par with Supreme Court Justices. Comparison with earlier studies indicates a definite, though small, increase in prestige from 1925 until the late forties at least. C. Wright Mills' study of class in a middle-sized city in the mid-forties indicated that with respect to their class origins, marriages, education, and job histories, "the free professionals [doctors and lawyers] are similar to the big business owners and executives" rather than to the small businessmen whose incomes they more closely approximate. The society pages of newspapers indicate the social acceptability of doctors as husbands to the daughters of the wealthy. G. William Domhoff's 1967 study of adult males listed in the *Social Register* (a guide to high society that represents the upper stratum of the upper class) revealed that no less than 8 percent of the adult males listed had the title "doctor" (presumably in almost all cases, MDs). This is a fifteen-fold overrepresentation: doctors make up only about 0.55 percent of the adult male population as a whole. And a quick look at magazines aimed at doctors, such as *Medical Economics*, conveys a vivid impression of upper- and upper-middle-class lifestyles—country clubs, travel, heavy stock market involvement, etc. [19]

Whether we look at class origin, present incomes, assets, lifestyles, or patterns of social interaction, we are on safe grounds in saying that doctors are generally members of the American upper

58 *Barbara and John Ehrenreich*

and upper-middle classes. Relative to the overwhelming majority of patients whether poor, "working class," or "middle class," they are distinctly upper class.

THE CONTENT OF COOPTATIVE SOCIAL CONTROL BY THE MEDICAL SYSTEM TODAY

We have noted two major developments in the medical system since 1930: (1) an expansion of services in several dimensions, accompanied by a broadening and deepening public dependency on the medical system; (2) the lack of a proportional expansion in the numbers of the chief functionaries of the medical system, the doctors, accompanied by an absolute and relative improvement in the social position of doctors. Within the medical system, doctors remain the unquestioned elite, holding a monopoly on the key functions of diagnosis, defining of illness, management of illness, and communications with patients. Within the larger society, doctors are also an elite group, members of the politically, economically, and culturally dominant strata. We can now put these two developments together: the expanding public dependency on the medical system is a dependency on *white, upper-middle- or upper-class males*.

To put it another way: the expansion of services and of utilization means that more people have more contacts with socially advantaged white male professionals, over more "needs" and "problems," than ever before. What is the nature of these contacts? What is the character of the social relationships that arise? The outstanding features of the doctor-patient relationship as a social interaction are:

1. *Intimacy*. Patients are required to expose their bodies to detailed visual and manual probing, and to confide their deepest anxieties about their physical condition. In addition, the patient is usually urged to confide in the doctor about other personal matters that may be peripheral to the problem at hand—family relations, sexual relations, the use of drugs or alcohol, etc. The intimacy, of course, goes only one way: doctors do not confide in their patients, nor do they undress. "Intimate" revelations may, of course, be essential to proper diagnosis and treatment. For our

purposes, it is important to note that intimacy and personal trust cannot readily be restricted to the narrow imperatives of a particular episode of disease. Parsons has argued (correctly, we think) that

> through processes which are mostly unconscious the physician tends to acquire various types of projective significance as a person which may not be directly relevant to his specifically technical functions. . . . The generally accepted name for this phenomenon in psychiatric circles is "transference," the attribution to the physician of significances to the patient which are not "appropriate" to the realistic situation, but which derive from the psychological needs of the patient. For understandable reasons a particularly important class of these involves the attributes of parental role as experienced by the patient in childhood. . . . [Thus] the situation of medical practice is such as inevitably to "involve" the physician in the psychologically significant "private" affairs of his patients.[20]

2. *Authority.* Patients are required to submit to the medical management of their problems almost without question. The penalty for excessive questioning is usually a quick put-down— "Where did *you* go to medical school?" "What are you so anxious about?" (Anxiety is in itself pathological, so this rejoinder amounts to the diagnosis of a new illness.) And so on. The penalties for persistent questioning, outright criticism, or general uncooperativeness are more severe: first, the doctor may reject the patient—"You'll have to find someone else." (Sometimes the rejection is accompanied by dire warnings. For example, a doctor once rejected one of the writers, for questioning the necessity of further lab tests, with the statement, "I don't care if you die!" Fortunately, the condition was far from life-threatening.) Finally, the doctor may "blacklist" the patient among other doctors whom he knows or works with. But these penalties need seldom be invoked: most patients accept the authoritarianism of the doctor and would be bewildered or even let down by more egalitarian treatment. What is especially interesting for our purposes is that the authoritarianism of the doctor-patient relationship increases as the social distance between doctor and patient increases. The degree of authoritarianism is greater for poor and working-class patients, nonwhite patients, female patients; and, as the class

position of doctors advances, it becomes greater for everyone else, too.

It should be stressed that these features of the doctor-patient relationship do not apply only to doctors and "sick" patients; people seeking preventive care, prenatal care, contraceptives or abortions, or cosmetic surgery all experience intimate and authoritarian relationships with doctors. To a lesser degree, so do people who are only indirectly involved in the encounter— parents of children needing care, children of aged parents. To enter a situation of professional dominance, you do not have to enter a sick role. In fact, you do not even have to be a patient.

Why do people submit to—in fact, struggle for access to—this kind of relationship, given that it is characterized by a degree of intimacy and authority that would be considered humiliating in any other social relationship? The obvious answer is that people expect to get immediate relief or help, and very often this expectation is met. There are effective contraceptives, antibiotics, surgical interventions, and so on. Cutting through the inflated advertising of medical miracles, and even correcting for iatrogenic effects, there *is* a valid body of biomedical technology, and the only available route to it is through a relationship of professional dominance. But, quite apart from the technology, the relationship itself has a kind of therapeutic value: if the doctor cannot solve your problem—and in a society characterized by insidious chronic disorders, the likelihood is that he cannot "solve" it—he can at least manage it. The therapeutic value of professional dominance, from the patient's point of view, is that the problem becomes the *doctor's* problem. It is not for you to fret or question the treatment; it's in the doctor's hands now and "he ought to know what he's doing." The authoritarianism of the relationship fosters a magical transference of the problem from patient to doctor. (This transference phenomenon, not to be confused with the kind of transference that Parsons discusses, is probably related to the inability of American medicine to deal adequately with problems that require the patient's willed participation in the cure—e.g., by giving up smoking. Patients expect to be cured, or at least to gain legitimate exemptions from work; they do not expect the doctor to impose new hardships.)

There are some crude similarities between the relationship of professional dominance and other relationships people enter into with powerful, socially advantaged others. Authoritarianism, rewards for submission, penalties for disobedience, and even "magical transference" ("I wouldn't want to be boss—or president, or foreman—think of all the responsibility") are common to such relationships. But the relationship that one has with a doctor is also profoundly different from any other relationship that one is likely to have with an authority figure, especially one who is of such elevated social class. It is a uniquely intimate and personal relationship. How many other important people are interested in you and concerned about you, even if only for a few minutes each month or year? And it is a manifestly benevolent relationship: disobeying a teacher or boss might be seen as gutsy, but disobeying a doctor can only be construed as irrational.

To backtrack a little: we have said that an expansionary medical system is characterized by cooptative social control. In order to understand the ideological nature of that control, we have examined the social relationships required for the delivery of medical care. These are relationships of intimate dominance by a professional elite consisting overwhelmingly of white, upper- and upper-middle-class males. These relationships are tolerated, in fact sought after, for their technologically and psychologically therapeutic effects. It should be evident that such relationships, often bridging the most powerful and the least powerful social groups, are rich in possibilities for social control: first, they are ideal vehicles for the transmission of ideological messages from the socially dominant group, and we shall consider this possibility in a moment. But at least as important, it seems to us, is the ideological impact of the relationship itself. A relationship of dominance and dependency, of intimacy and authority, between a person and a member of the upper class can only act *to promote acquiescence to a social system built on class- and sex-based inequalities in power.*

There is no conspiracy behind this. But neither is it true that ideological control of this type is a natural and inevitable concomitant of the delivery of medical services. It is possible—in fact it is easy—to imagine a highly technologically advanced medi-

cal system which engenders a very different sort of social relationship—one in which sickness is not an occasion for isolation of the individual or for his or her subjection to medical "management," but for collective concern and mutual assistance; one in which the experience of the patient is not self-alienation but self-help; one in which helping roles are occupied by social equals, and being helped has no stigma of submission. Of course, such a system would still be exerting social control, but in an entirely different ideological direction—one of self-determination, and solidarity among equals.

Perhaps we can generalize and state that the social mechanisms which arise in any society for the care of dependent persons—children, the aged, the handicapped, the ill—must always operate in the direction of social cohesion. (In fact, the existence of such mechanisms is one of the defining characteristics of a "society.") The question is, cohesion to whom, to what groups? In pretechnological situations, the social mechanisms for illness and other forms of dependency commonly involve the formation or tightening of bonds between individuals of similar social status—local midwife and pregnant women, grandmother and sick child, etc. In particular, such relationships often centered in and helped strengthen the family. By contrast, the situation in the United States is that not only disease, but also a growing number of other conditions, call for the formation of primary social bonds to members of the upper classes. The effect is certainly to promote social cohesion, only in this case it is cohesion between social groups whose ultimate interests are not the same.[21]

There is another aspect of cooptative social control that we have alluded to: the use of the doctor-patient relationship for the transmission of overt ideological messages. This is probably the most familiar type of social control exercised by the medical system—the racist and sexist put-downs, digs about a patient's lifestyle, etc.—but it is extremely difficult to pin down or document. The well-known confidentiality of the doctor-patient relationship (which is essential for the intimacy) has precluded any systematic studies of the social interaction that goes on. Furthermore, some of the most interesting ideological messages

probably come through thoroughly disguised as technical directives or advice. All we can do here is to give some examples of the types of messages communicated by doctors, without attempting to establish their prevalence or impact. We distinguish three broad types of messages:

1. Messages that are completely unrelated to the technical requirements of the encounter. This would include comments by the doctor on elections, legislation, or any other broad public issues. Although this use of a doctor's time may seem highly improbable to those of us unaccustomed to clinic care, it is apparently not that unusual. AM-PAC (the AMA's Political Action Committee) unabashedly recommends that doctors make good use of their working hours to inform patients about public issues and candidates.[22] In the AMA's all-out fight against Medicare and pro-Medicare political candidates a few years ago, doctors resorted to such tactics as putting political flyers in with their bills, lecturing their patients before healing them, and threatening to drop politically uncongenial patients.[23]

2. Messages that are related to the technical aspects of the encounter, but that are patently gratuitous. For example, a black woman whom we know complained of weakness and tiredness; she was told by the doctor that "colored people are always lazy." Most of our knowledge about this kind of message comes from the women's movement, in which women have made a point of sharing with each other their experiences with doctors. Again, we can only be anecdotal. One woman had a doctor tell her that her breasts were "too small," and then say, "Oh well, as long as your husband is satisfied . . ." Another woman, a teacher, was advised to douche every day because "professional women should always douche." In addition to these kinds of messages, which have the obvious effect of reinforcing the patient's sense of sexual or racial inferiority, doctors also transmit a great deal of conventional morality on such subjects as sex and drugs. In fact, some parents rely on the doctor to introduce their teenagers to these subjects. Doctors are important arbiters of what is moral (usually represented as what is "normal") in sexual activity, drug use, and drinking.

3. Messages disguised as technical communications. This cat-

egory is potentially limitless. Who, especially among lay people, is able to distinguish between technically necessary and relevant communications and covert social opinions? For example, women's self-help groups report that a great many women are told that their uteruses are "tipped"—an apparently neutral observation which, by suggesting abnormalities of reproductive function, invariably has the effect of reinforcing feelings of inadequacy. However, in their own work, the self-help groups have discovered that most uteruses are tipped to one degree or another, including those of women who have successfully borne children. To take another case, pediatricians frequently counsel parents (in books written for the public as well as in office communications) not to put small children in day-care centers on the grounds that the children will catch too many infectious diseases. This advice obviously acts to discourage mothers from working, but it is scientifically unfounded: there are no studies in the English language medical literature showing significantly higher morbidity among children in day-care centers.[24] More generally, the actual treatment given by doctors to poor patients may differ from that given to middle-class and wealthy patients. One form of medical care, psychiatric treatment, is known to vary with class—the more affluent patients get psychotherapy while the less affluent are more likely to be treated with drugs. And differential attitudes of doctors toward patients of different socioeconomic class have been documented. There are certainly grounds for speculation, at least, that the actual technical medical treatment of the poor may be a factor in strengthening the feelings of "low self-worth" which many sociologists claim to detect in the poor—i.e., that the medical system reinforces the sense of class inferiority in those of lower class position when they use its services.

The point is that the doctor-patient relationship is an ideal one for the transmission of almost any kind of message that doctors may feel inclined to convey. Given the intimacy and authoritarianism built into the relationship, and the prestige and presumed expertise of the doctor, the patient is likely to take such messages much more seriously than he or she would from other people. Whether there is any consistent content to these medical messages is a matter for further investigation. Certainly in the

case of women's medical care there seems to be consistent bias toward sexism. It is tempting to speculate that medical messages in general may consistently reflect the attitudes of the social group to which doctors belong. If so, we would have to regard the medical system as a significant vehicle of communication between the upper classes and the general public.[25]

CLASS DIFFERENCES IN THE SOCIAL CONTROL IMPACT
OF THE MEDICAL SYSTEM

We have spent so much time analyzing the nature of the cooptative control exerted by the medical system because the expansionary nature of the present system makes this kind of control more important than it has been at any other time in our history. But disciplinary social control is still an extremely important social factor. The two kinds of control—cooptative and disciplinary—affect different groups of people in different ways and in different proportions. In fact, the exact mix of cooptative and disciplinary control experienced by different groups has been changing very rapidly. The result of these changes has been in many cases the very opposite of "social control"—public dissatisfaction and even upheaval.

We will confine our discussion to two very broad economic groups, largely omitting the dimensions of age, sex, and race. (1) The first group is what we will call the "medical poor"—people who are "medically indigent" though not necessarily on Medicaid or welfare. In the big cities, this group is made up predominately of nonwhites and the elderly of all races. Their major sources of care are institutional—hospital wards, clinics, and emergency rooms. (2) The second group is what we will call the "medical middle class"—people who are not medically indigent but who feel the effects of rapidly rising medical costs. Their major source of primary care is the private physician in group or solo practice.[26] (Above these two groups are wealthier groups who do not concern us as subjects of social control. They experience no barriers to medical care and, in fact, form the market for luxury care. They are in roughly the same social classes as physicians.)

The medical poor. Historically the poor and the near-poor were

simply excluded from the medical system by their inability to pay. Even in urban areas where charity services were available, the poor showed considerably lower utilization rates than middle-class people—a difference made all the more striking by the fact that the poor have always had much higher *disease* rates than other groups. Utilization by the poor picked up somewhat in the sixties but there remain serious gaps: the black poor underutilize services even when they are free or financed by Medicaid, and the poor of all ethnic groups underutilize preventive services (immunizations, annual check-ups, cancer screening, etc.), again, even when these services are free.[27] To explain the persistence of underutilization even after financial barriers are removed, it has become fashionable to invoke a peculiar mind-set among the poor—they lack "future orientation," or they regard their bodies as machines "to be worn out but not repaired";[28] they are "alienated" or poorly "integrated" socially.[29]

A far simpler, though less comforting, explanation is that most of the services available to the poor are so unappealing that they actively discourage utilization. The picture of the bottom half of the two-class medical system has been painted often enough—the decaying public health centers presided over by equally decaying municipal doctors, the crowded clinic waiting rooms patrolled by security guards, the open wards with twenty or more beds staffed by a single practical nurse, and in some cases an active contingent of vermin—and so on. Medicaid or no, such services are a painful deterrent to getting sick, and even to seeking the care that should prevent sickness. We would say that the services for the poor are constructed, wittingly or unwittingly, to exercise disciplinary social control.[30]

But there has been, in the last ten years, a significant expansion of services for the poor beyond the traditional clinic/ward type. This expansion has brought the poor, for the first time, into the sphere of cooptative social control by the medical system. In addition to the general class-bridging effects discussed above, cooptative control has taken some very specific and overt forms in the case of the poor. Consider the forms which this expansion of services has taken:

First, health services for the poor have not expanded uni-

formly. Certain specialized services, particularly birth control and out-patient mental health services, have expanded out of proportion to the expansion of general health services. For many ghetto residents, a simple infection still means a grim day spent at a hospital clinic, while for problems of fecundity or psychoneurosis there may be well-appointed centers equipped with interpreters, outreach workers, and baby-sitting services. This disproportionate concern with birth control and mental hygiene has been directly interpreted in Third World communities as a social control effort. Black militants have denounced ghetto birth control services as "genocidal," and have suggested that the mental health services represent a refined police surveillance system. Whether one considers birth control and mental health services to be desirable or not, it is clear that they do have the alleged effects—reduction of birth rates and more efficient detection of social deviants.

Second, there has been some expansion of general medical services in the form of comprehensive medical centers—government-financed group practices for the poor. These "neighborhood" or "community" health centers, as they are called, were designed to provide the poor with the kind of personal, continuous relationships with doctors which do not usually occur in the clinic setting. To the extent that this aim has been met (and it should be pointed out that many community health centers are little more than small-scale versions of the impersonal clinics in the sponsoring hospital), the community health centers are settings for the cooptative control of the poor as individuals, bringing them into relationships of professional dominance. In addition, the community health centers in many cases represented an attempt to control the poor *collectively*. At the most obvious level, many centers were created with the explicitly cooptative aim of cooling out a hostile community. The Watts community gained a center a year after the 1965 riot, and countless "Martin Luther King Health Centers" dot the land.

The community health centers also exert direct community control in an even more conventional sense. As institutions with budgets ranging from $2 million on up, they are often the most important economic centers in their localities. They have be-

come, in many cases, key centers of political patronage, offering scores of unskilled and semiskilled jobs to the friends of local power brokers (Democratic Party heavies, OEO officials, and a whole raft of other minor bosses resentfully termed "poverty pimps"). For example, the Hunts Point Multi-Service Center in the South Bronx—a health center *cum* housing, legal, and social services—was the launching pad for Democratic city councilman and local party boss Ramon Velez.[31] His center, and dozens like it, have served as nuclei for the reconstruction of Democratic machines in the cities. It seems likely that this was the conscious intent of the Democratic administrations of the sixties when they designed that cornucopia of scant services and lush patronage called the "War on Poverty."[32]

On a less obvious level, the community health centers have had a *culturally* destructive effect. Fanon might have described them as outposts of the white man's culture planted in "the colonies" to undermine the cultural identity of the oppressed. Whether or not this was the intent, it was probably an important effect. The black, Puerto Rican, and Chicano target populations of most centers have (or did have) rich traditions of folk medicine which were integral to community structure—*curanderos*, botanical healers, spiritualists, not to mention skilled aunts and grandmothers. If professional medicine was to make significant inroads, it was essential that the community health centers discredit, destroy, or coopt the prevailing folkways. The doctors worked on this directly, and the most ambitiously cooptative centers employed anthropologists and other social scientists to assist them.

Professionals in the community health centers "movement" often felt themselves working uphill against community resistance or indifference. Underutilization was a widespread problem, especially in the early years. Accustomed to an exclusionary medical system, poor people tended to view these new expansionary enterprises with suspicion. Ever more cooptative tactics were employed to "win the hearts and minds of the people": the employment of local people to do outreach work, the addition of training programs for semiprofessional medical jobs, the creation of community advisory boards. (In the view of many medical

progressives, such methods were not only appealing come-ons; they were therapeutic in themselves, helping to break through the "social pathology" of the ghetto.) The most ambitious and "sensitive" centers presented uniformly black or brown faces to the community (though the doctors and directors were still white); they virtually dragnetted their catchment areas for patients; they sent out trained community workers to track down appointment-breakers. The result, in a number of cases, was soon *overutilization*, and with it a rapid decay of the amenities which had distinguished these centers from mere clinics.

With the community health center movement, the advertising of professional medicine far exceeded its ability to deliver. Federal funds began to wane as early as 1968, and few doctors have enough Schweitzer in them to enter grantless ghettos. But, as is well known by now, expectations had been raised. If there was a life-giving center for Watts, why not for Hough, or south Chicago, or Bedford-Stuyvesant? In fact, the same may be said for all the tentative expansions of the medical system into the ghettos. To the extent that they did touch the hearts and the minds of the people, they raised dangerous and unmeetable expectations. If mental health meant peace of mind, then why didn't the community mental health center do something about slum landlords? If the hospital and its outreach center stood for health, what were they doing about garbage in the streets? In the end, the medical approach to the problems of the ghetto succeeded only in putting the heat on the medical institutions of the ghetto—for *all* of the problems of the ghetto.

The medical middle class. It is this group, far more than the poor, that experienced the medical expansion of the forties through sixties. Here we find the fastest-rising utilization rates and the skyrocketing expenditures. Health insurance, whether in the form of a hard-won fringe benefit or an expensive private purchase, has made the increased consumption possible. Rising expectations have made it necessary. Members of this group, both blue- and white-collar, are better educated than ever before, more attuned to the benefits of technology, more accepting of professional expertise. And it is here that we find the TV medical drama viewers, the readers of doctor novels, diet books, and sex

manuals. Here are the weight-watchers and cholesterol watchers—anxious about the seven earliest signs of cancer, and anxious about anxiety itself. Here, much more than among the poor today or the working class of a generation ago, it is expected that birth, death, and any extremes of experience (pain, madness) will be overseen by physicians and sequestered in institutions. There are scattered pockets of cultural resistance—to mental health services among older blue-collar people, to family limitation services among some Catholic groups—but these are largely vestigial. The general orientation has been to rush headlong into the expanding medical system with whatever money one has, and get as much as one can take.

However, there is a very serious and growing exclusionary trend countering this rush to consumption. We have already emphasized the failure of the medical profession to expand numerically in proportion to the demand for medical services. For our medical middle class, this does not yet mean that doctors themselves are in short supply, but it does mean that doctors' *time* is getting scarce. Private practitioners have been increasing their patient loads without proportionately increasing their working time. For the individual patient, this means longer waits for appointments (four to six weeks is not unusual for a specialist), longer waiting times at the office, shorter, more impersonal encounters with the doctor, and, of course, no house calls at all. One may well ask what is left of the celebrated doctor-patient relationship when ten or fifteen minutes is allotted per patient and part of this time is spent with a nurse or medical assistant who takes histories, weighs the patient, gives instructions on prescribed regimens, etc. The suburban doctor's office is becoming no less an impersonal mill than the urban out-patient clinic.[33]

With the exclusionary trends in the care received by the medical middle class, disciplinary social control comes into operation. Long waits and frustrating encounters with doctors lead to the common feeling that "I don't want to bother the doctor." Even in the more educated strata, people are not fully utilizing preventive services such as Pap tests, breast exams, and vaccinations, nor are they reliably bringing the "first signs" of various diseases to medical attention. From a public health point of view, the results are

discouraging: diseases that are preventable or curable if caught early continue to be major killers. But people are only responding to the clear message *not* to bother the doctor—to keep on the job.[34]

There is every indication that the exclusionary trends in the care received by the medical middle class are the wave of the future. In fact, it is government policy to augment them, but by different means. "HMOs" (Health Maintenance Organizations) and "PSROs" (Professional Standards Review Organizations)—widely misinterpreted as consumer "victories"—are actually devices to reduce medical expenditures by reducing utilization of medical services.[35] HMOs sound like an expansion of services, something like community health centers for the medical middle class. In reality they are financial arrangements to provide participating doctors with incentives to curb utilization (particularly of expensive hospital services). HMOs can, in fact, substantially reduce costs without lowering the overall quality of care provided. But the HMO financial arrangement has the potential, at least, to permit doctors to profit personally from excessive underutilization; fragmentary evidence suggests that this may have happened in some HMOs.[36] PSROs sound like an effort to make doctors accountable to the public by forcing them to monitor each others' services. But the only thing that will really be monitored is utilization (was this lab test or this hospital admission really necessary, etc.)—not quality. These reforms are efforts to discipline the demanding public, with the doctors serving as the disciplinary agents.

CONCLUSION

In the last section we have attempted to dissect the uneasy mix of expansionary and exclusionary tendencies in people's medical experience. We have endeavored to show that both tendencies, both types of systems, exert social control and operate to maintain the status quo.

The exclusionary and expansionary tendencies arise in part from the internal dynamics of the medical system, but, as should be apparent to anyone who follows public policy in health, they

are also shaped by the overt intervention of the ruling class. One element of the ruling class—the one that held sway over public policy during the Kennedy and Johnson years—is expansionist, and favors increased public spending to promote further expansion. The other, which was represented by the Nixon Administration, is exclusionary and favors government intervention to curb what are viewed as the "excesses" of the sixties.

The two groups are, of course, the groups usually distinguished as the "liberal" and "conservative" elements of the ruling class. Their different approaches to the medical system mirror their approaches to social control in general. The liberals, for example, favor rehabilitation of criminals, medical care for addicts, and less authoritarian structures of work and education. The conservatives favor punitive treatment of criminals, addicts, and other deviants, and even more authoritarianism in the family, the job, and the schools. One group seeks to manage discontent through cooptation; the other through repression. One believes that the structure of society can be held together by ideological persuasion: the other puts its trust ultimately only in force. To repeat what is almost a truism, but represents a central radical understanding of the sixties: neither group is about to remove the fundamental inequities that are the sources of discontent. And neither group trusts the people to be unmanipulated and unpoliced—nor have they any reason to.

On the whole, the radical approach to health has been little more than an amplified echo of the liberal, expansionist faction of the ruling class. Radicals have simply demanded that medical services be more readily available to all, with the qualification that the services should represent technically high-quality care, delivered with dignity and without racism or sexism.

It is time that we transcended the argument in these terms. It is time that we got off the single axis of "more" or "less" and began to ask "more" of what, for what purpose, to what effect? The only way to do this is to free *ourselves* from the medical mystification that confines us to seeing medical care as something wholly ordained by technology—a "commodity" whose social nature cannot be examined because it is believed to have none.[37]

We have tried to make a start in this direction. But the more

serious tasks lie ahead. If the medical system is understood as something more than a system for distributing a "commodity," if it is understood as a system of direct *social relationships*, then the question becomes: what kinds of social relationships do we want a medical system to foster? How can we design a system so that the social relationships that it engenders promote *socialist* relationships in society in general?

The task that we are posing is not just an exercise in utopian engineering. It is not the same as asking how one would design an electrical power system under socialism, or how one would manage the water supply. The medical system itself has deluded us into thinking that the problems addressed by medicine are indeed "medical" or "technical" problems—that they are properly the preserve of specialists and experts who stand outside culture and politics. But the problems which our society relegates to the medical system—the care of the disabled and dependent, the management of reproduction, individual suffering, and death—are no less than some of the central problems which confront any human society. Medicine has allowed us to evade them too long.

NOTES

1. The most complete radical treatment of the health system are Barbara and John Ehrenreich, *The American Health Empire* (A Health-PAC Book) (New York: Random House, 1970); *Billions for Bandaids*, ed. T. Bodenheimer, S. Cummings, and E. Harding (San Francisco: Medical Committee for Human Rights, 1972); *Prognosis Negative: Crisis in the Health Care System*, ed. David Kotelchuck (A Health-PAC Book; New York: Vintage, 1976); Vicente Navarro, *Medicine Under Capitalism* (New York: Prodist, 1976).
2. *Going Crazy*, ed. H. M. Ruitenbeck (New York: Bantam Books, 1972); and P. Chesler, *Women and Madness* (New York: Avon, 1972).
3. Boston Women's Health Collective, *Our Bodies, Ourselves* (New York: Simon & Schuster, 1972); and *Health-PAC Bulletin*, (May 1970).
4. Talcott Parsons, *The Social System* (New York: Free Press, 1951), pp. 428-79; Eliot Freidson, *The Profession of Medicine* (New York: Dodd Mead & Co., 1970) esp. pp. 203-331; Talcott Parsons, "Definitions of Health and Illness in the Light of American Values and

Social Structure," in *Patients, Physicians and Illness*, ed. E. Gartly Jao, 2nd ed. (New York: Free Press, 1972), p. 107.

5. Parsons, *The Social System*, pp. 118, 121. In Parsons' scheme, sickness poses something of a moral dilemma to American society which, he argues, has an unusually high regard for health and activism. For humanitarian reasons, we feel obliged to treat the sick well—but never so well, or so visibly well, that others will be tempted to seek the same treatment by joining the ranks of the "sick." One may wonder why a people who supposedly value activism and work so highly find sickness so alluring. Could they possibly be *oppressed* and feel that, in Parsons' words, "the way to deal with the frustrating aspects of the social system is 'for everybody to get sick' " (Parsons, *The Social System*, p. 477)? But oppression is not a dimension of Parsons' analysis. Borrowing from psychoanalytic theory, Parsons explains this anomaly in terms of American patterns of child-raising.

6. Frances Fox Piven and Richard A. Cloward, *Regulating the Poor* (New York: Pantheon, 1971), pp. 33-36.

7. Freidson, *Profession of Medicine*, p. 304.

8. Ibid., pp. 329, 330.

9. Philip Rieff, *Freud: The Mind of the Novelist* (Garden City: Doubleday, 1961), p. 360, cited in Freidson, *Profession of Medicine*, p. 248.

10. Freidson, *Profession of Medicine*, p. 250.

11. A concept advanced by the Health Policy Advisory Center to describe the increasing centralization of urban medical services around medical schools and major teaching hospitals. Strictly speaking, an "empire" would include the core controlling institution (medical school or teaching hospital) plus all its affiliated lesser hospitals and health centers of various types. Usually, though, the word "empire" has been used in reference to the core institution only. See *The American Health Empire*, chapters 3-6.

12. Michel Foucault, *Madness and Civilization* (New York: Pantheon, 1965), pp. 46-64.

13. See B. Ehrenreich and D. English, *Complaints and Disorders: The Sexual Politics of Sickness* (Old Westbury, N.Y.: Feminist Press, 1973); excerpts appear in this volume.

14. Per capita expenditures on health services and supplies, adjusted for the increase in the medical care component of the consumer price index, rose (in 1970 dollars) from $169.92 in 1950 to $315.83 in 1970, an 86 percent increase. This represented a jump from 4.6 percent of GNP to 7.1 percent. Utilization of virtually all kinds of services has risen rapidly, although not entirely synchronously for all types.

Out-of-hospital utilization of doctors rose from 2.6 visits per person per annum in 1928-31 to 4.7 per annum in 1958-59 and has stayed at about that level ever since. Hospital out-patient visits per capita increased 66 percent from 1962 to 1970 alone (541 visits per 1000 population to 899 visits per 1000 population). Out-patient psychiatric services (community mental health centers, day treatment services, clinics) increased 34.4 percent from 1955 to 1969 (2.3 visits/1000 population to 10.2 visits/1000).

Utilization of in-patient services has also increased sharply: annual general hospital admissions and mental hospital admissions per 1000 population more than doubled between 1940 and 1970 (general hospitals: 74 per 1000 population per annum to 152 per 1000; mental hospitals: 1.4 per 1000 to 3.3 per 1000). The population of nursing homes increased from 491,000 to 850,000 (94 percent) from 1963 to 1969. (All data from *Statistical Abstract of the U.S.*, 1972, except physician utilization for 1928-31 cited in Odin W. Anderson and Ronald M. Anderson, "Patterns of Use of Health Services," in *Handbook of Medical Sociology*, ed. H. E. Freeman et al. (Englewood Cliffs, N.J.: Prentice-Hall, 1972).

15. It is not, strictly speaking, the technology itself which inflates expectations, but the *advertising* of the technology. In the popular family and women's magazines, health and medical articles probably outnumber those on any other subject except marriage: "Researchers Claim New Pill Will Ease Tension Without Side Effects," "What You Should Know About Stomach Aches," etc. (A journal aimed at doctors recently ran a drug company ad for a new low-estrogen oral contraceptive: "Because her 'medical journals' alarm her about 'the pill' . . . and because she runs to you for her answer . . ." (*Medical World News*, January 11, 1974). Or look at TV: in a recent week in New York City, there were ten weekly shows, two daily shows, and two "specials" concerned with doctors or medicine, a total of fourteen hours of programming. The media both feed on and fan the public's fascination with medicine.

16. U.S. Bureau of the Census, *Historical Statistics of the United States, Colonial Times to 1957*; see also Rosemary Stevens, *American Medicine and the Public Interest* (New Haven: Yale University Press, 1971) for the full story of the turn-of-the-century reforms.

17. Occupational figures from R. Fein and G. Weber, *The Financing of Medical Education* (New York: McGraw-Hill, 1970); percentages of women and blacks from U.S. Bureau of the Census, *Statistical Abstract of the United States*, 1972.

18. Income figures from *Historical Statistics of the United States, Colo-*

nial *Times to* 1957 and *Statistical Abstract of the United States*, 1972; asset figures cited in Fein and Weber, *Financing of Medical Education*.
19. R. W. Hodge, P. M. Siegel, and P. H. Rossi, "Occupational Prestige in the United States, 1925-63," *American Journal of Sociology* 70 (1964): 286–302; C. Wright Mills, "The Middle Classes in Middle-Sized Cities," in C. Wright Mills, *Power, Politics and People* (New York: Oxford, 1967); G. William Domhoff, *Who Rules America?* (Englewood Cliffs, N.J.: Prentice-Hall, 1967).
20. Parsons, *The Social System*, p. 453.
21. In at least one country that is seeking to develop a technically modern medical system, China, the state has made it a conscious policy to diminish the social distance between medical personnel and the people. In China, we would suggest, the social organization of medicine operates to promote cohesion within the working classes and the nation. See Joshua Horn, *Away with All Pests* (New York: Monthly Review Press, 1970).
22. "How the Opinion Maker Makes Opinion in Politics," leaflet from the American Medical Political Action Committee (c. 1973).
23. Richard Harris, *A Sacred Trust* (Baltimore: Penguin, 1969).
24. Based on a review of the *Cumulative Index Medicus*, the standard index of medical literature, for the years 1963-1973 inclusive.
25. There are several reasons to hypothesize a consistent, class-oriented content:

    1. The intense socialization of doctors as students and interns and residents probably produces a certain uniformity of attitudes. It is interesting that certain features of their socialization—repeated sleeplessness and interrogations—resemble the supposed "brainwashing" of POWs.

    2. At least *moral* uniformity is rigidly imposed on practicing doctors by a system of peer surveillance which doctors would find intolerable if applied to their technical performance.

    3. The AMA provides doctors with pamphlets, lecture outlines, and the like, offering, at least, to "think" for the busy doctor on a variety of social issues.

    4. Doctors are fairly uniformly upper-middle or upper class. Especially in smaller cities, they are members of the local ruling class, associating with local businessmen, bankers, lawyers, etc. and presumably sharing moral and political attitudes with them.
26. Note: These broad categories gloss over some important differences in medical experience. Among the poor, there are major differences

between the young and the elderly, the urban and the rural, and probably between the working poor and welfare recipients. In the "medical middle" we should probably distinguish between a poorer and less urban group receiving most of its care from GPs and a more prosperous, urban group which is plugged into the network of specialists.

The working class includes both the "medical poor" and part of the "medical middle class." (Many members of the petty bourgeoisie and professional-managerial class are in the latter group, as well.) The division of the working class into two components reflects the complex internal stratification of the working class, which, in terms of medical care as well as of many other criteria, is not homogeneous. The impact of different patterns of medical care for different sectors of the working class in *maintaining* the internal stratification of the class remains to be explored more thoroughly.

27. William C. Richardson, "Poverty, Illness and the Use of Health Services in the United States," in Jaco, *Patients, Physicians, and Illness*, pp. 240–49; Anderson and Anderson, "Patterns of Use of Health Services"; Rashi Fein, *The Doctor Shortage: An Economic Diagnosis* (Washington, D.C.: Brookings Institution, 1967).
28. Daniel Rosenblatt and Edward A. Suchman, "The Underutilization of Medical-Care Services by Blue-Collarites," in *Blue-Collar World*, ed. Arthur B. Shostak and William Gomberg (Englewood Cliffs, N.J.: Prentice-Hall, 1964).
29. Philip M. Moody and Robert M. Gray, "Social Class, Social Integration, and the Use of Preventive Health Services," in Jaco, *Patients, Physicians, and Illness*, pp. 250–61.
30. Other immediate sources of underutilization of services include the costs of transportation and of taking time off from work, inconveniently located services, racism and simple rudeness from hospital workers, maintenance of "folk healing" traditions, and lack of knowledge about health facilities and about health itself.

More fundamentally, it is notable that this one segment of the working class is excluded from medical care far more often than other segments. The reasons for this, we would speculate, lie in part, at least, in the lower value that our society places on the lives of economically marginally productive people, and in part on the "need" to instill values of "industrial" work discipline in peoples of more recent rural origin (as many urban slum dwellers are).
31. *New York Times*, November 19, 1973, p. 37.
32. See Piven and Cloward, *Regulating the Poor*, pp. 250–84.

33. In the large and reputedly "excellent" suburban group practice that we use, an affiliate of New York's Health Insurance Plan, ten minutes are allotted for each pediatric and gynecological visit, and the time for annual check-ups has recently been cut from thirty minutes to fifteen minutes.

34. A very significant medical tendency which we suspect is related to the time pressure on the private practitioner is the diagnosis of physical complaints as psychosomatic. The evidence for this is indirect, but impressive: (1) Private practitioners themselves commonly estimate that at least 50 percent of the cases they see are "psychosomatic." (2) Studies of prescribing habits of doctors show that tranquilizers are the most commonly prescribed drug. A psychosomatic diagnosis—medically accurate or not—clearly amounts to a diagnosis of *malingering*.

35. Both HMOs and PSROs are the children of Nixon Administration legislation. The former are provided for in the Health Maintenance Organization Act of 1973 and the latter in the Social Security Act Amendments of 1972. The immediate origins of both programs are in government concern over the fantastically rapid rise in government health-care expenditures in the years since 1965. We are indebted to Harry Becker for our interpretation of these programs.

36. See, for instance, *Medical World News*, June 5, 1973, pp. 17–19; and the California Council for Health Plan Alternatives, "Evaluation Report" on the California Medical Group, prepared for Teamsters and Food Employers Security Trust Fund, Los Angeles (mimeo, 1972). Studies of the Kaiser plans have suggested that the HMO mechanism leads to sharp declines in the accessibility of services resulting in considerable tendencies for subscribers to the plans to seek out-of-plan care, in substantial differences in utilization by socioeconomic status, and so forth (see *Health-PAC Bulletin*, November 1973).

37. Equally, we must free ourselves from the economic mystification of health care, which confines us to seeing the health-care system as little more than a system through which doctors, drug companies, insurance companies, etc. extract profits from the sick. In this article we have ignored economic approaches to the medical system. Instead we have described the medical system as a system of social relationships. The economic and sociological approaches are not alternatives, but complementary. The economic approach can be used to explain the development of the medical system and to make predictions about its future development. This is because profits (or

at least the minimization of costs) are major motivations in the development of the system. But it cannot explain the *experience* of medical care, or the political implications of that experience for the larger social system. Conversely, the sociological approach that we have taken cannot explain the development of the medical system. The officials of the medical system are not motivated by a desire to exert ideological control in the interests of the larger capitalist system, and it would be ridiculous to imagine that they are. But the kind of approach that we have taken may help to point the way to an understanding of the cultural and political *impact* of the medical system on the larger society. And, though it may not help us to predict anything, it can help us to understand what kind of an ideological function a medical system might serve within a socialist society.

To say that the two approaches are complementary is to say that they must coexist in our understanding or else that understanding will be limited and superficial. A purely economic approach is often defended as the only "correct" Marxist approach. It is argued that the only Marxist understanding of capitalist society is an understanding in terms of the exchange of commodities. But it was Marx who insisted that under capitalism, the relationships between commodities, or between people and commodities, obscure and mystify the underlying relationships between people. We must not allow ourselves to be mystified *especially* when examining a sector of the economy in which the "commodity" is not a material thing but is in fact a direct human encounter.

The danger of the purely economic approach is not only that it leads to faulty analysis, but that it leads to a programmatic strategy which is basically economistic in nature. The only demand becomes "more"; the only challenge to capitalism is to produce "more" within the framework of an irrational and oppressive system.

IRVING KENNETH ZOLA

MEDICINE AS AN INSTITUTION
OF SOCIAL CONTROL

The theme of this essay is that medicine is becoming a major institution of social control, nudging aside, if not incorporating, the more traditional institutions of religion and law. It is becoming the new repository of truth, the place where absolute and often final judgments are made by supposedly morally neutral and objective experts. And these judgments are made, not in the name of virtue or legitimacy, but in the name of health. Moreover, this is not occurring through the political power physicians hold or can influence, but is largely an insidious and often undramatic phenomenon accomplished by "medicalizing" much of daily living, by making medicine and the labels "healthy" and "ill" *relevant* to an ever increasing part of human existence.

Although many have noted aspects of this process, by confining their concern to the field of psychiatry, these criticisms have been misplaced.[1] For psychiatry has by no means distorted the mandate of medicine, but indeed, though perhaps at a pace faster than other medical specialities, is following instead some of the basic claims and directions of that profession. Nor is this extension into society the result of any professional "imperialism," for this leads us to think of the issue in terms of misguided human

This paper was written while the author was a consultant in residence at the Netherlands Institute for Preventive Medicine, Leiden. For their general encouragement and the opportunity to pursue this topic I will always be grateful. It was presented at the Medical Sociology Conference of the British Sociological Association at Weston-super-Mare in November 1971. My special thanks for their extensive editorial and substantive comments go to Egon Bittner, Mara Sanadi, Alwyn Smith, and Bruce Wheaton.

efforts or motives. If we search for the "why" of this phenomenon, we will see instead that it is rooted in our increasingly
complex technological and bureaucratic system—a system which
has led us down the path of the reluctant reliance on the expert.[2]

Quite frankly, what is presented in the following pages is not a
definitive argument but rather a case in progress. As such it draws
heavily on observations made in the United States, though similar murmurings have long been echoed elsewhere.[3]

AN HISTORICAL PERSPECTIVE

The involvement of medicine in the management of society is
not new. It did not appear full-blown one day in the mid-
twentieth century. As Sigerist has aptly claimed,[4] medicine at
base was always not only a social science but an occupation
whose very practice was inextricably interwoven into society.
This interdependence is perhaps best seen in two branches of
medicine which have had a built-in social emphasis from the very
start—psychiatry[5] and public health/preventive medicine.[6] Public
health was always committed to changing social aspects of life—
from sanitary to housing to working conditions—and often used
the arm of the state (i.e., through laws and legal power) to gain its
ends (e.g., quarantines, vaccinations). Psychiatry's involvement
in society is a bit more difficult to trace, but taking the histories of
psychiatry as data, then one notes the almost universal reference
to one of the early pioneers, a physician named Johan Weyer.
His, and thus psychiatry's, involvement in social problems lay in
the objection that witches ought not to be burned; for they were
not possessed by the devil, but rather bedeviled by their
problems—namely they were insane. From its early concern with
the issue of insanity as a defense in criminal proceedings,
psychiatry has grown to become the most dominant rehabilitative
perspective in dealing with society's "legal" deviants. Psychiatry,
like public health, has also used the legal powers of the state in
the accomplishment of its goals (i.e., the cure of the patient)
through the legal proceedings of involuntary commitment and its
concomitant removal of certain rights and privileges.

This is not to say, however, that the rest of medicine has been

"socially" uninvolved. For a rereading of history makes it seem a matter of degree. Medicine has long had both a *de jure* and a *de facto* relation to institutions of social control. The *de jure* relationship is seen in the idea of reportable diseases, wherein, if certain phenomena occur in his practice, the physician is required to report them to the appropriate authorities. While this seems somewhat straightforward and even functional where certain highly contagious diseases are concerned, it is less clear where the possible spread of infection is not the primary issue (e.g., with gunshot wounds, attempted suicide, drug use and what is now called child abuse). The *de facto* relation to social control can be argued through a brief look at the disruptions of the last two or three American Medical Association conventions. For there the American Medical Association members—and really all ancillary health professions—were accused of practicing social control (the term used by the accusers was genocide) in, first, *whom* they have traditionally treated with *what*—giving *better* treatment to more favored clientele; and second, *what* they have treated—a more subtle form of discrimination in that, with limited resources, by focusing on some disease others are neglected. Here the accusation was that medicine has focused on the diseases of the rich and the established—cancer, heart disease, stroke—and ignored the diseases of the poor, such as malnutrition and still high infant mortality.

THE MYTH OF ACCOUNTABILITY

Even if we acknowledge such a growing medical involvement, it is easy to regard it as primarily a "good" one—which involves the steady destigmatization of many human and social problems. Thus Barbara Wootton was able to conclude:

> Without question . . . in the contemporary attitude toward antisocial behaviour, psychiatry and humanitarianism have marched hand in hand. Just because it is so much in keeping with the mental atmosphere of a scientifically-minded age, the medical treatment of social deviants has been a most powerful, perhaps even the most powerful, reinforcement of humanitarian impulses; for today the prestige of humane proposals is immensely enhanced if these are expressed in the idiom of medical science.[7]

The assumption is thus readily made that such medical involvement in social problems leads to their removal from religious and legal scrutiny and thus from moral and punitive consequences. In turn the problems are placed under medical and scientific scrutiny and thus in objective and therapeutic circumstances.

The fact that we cling to such a hope is at least partly due to two cultural-historical blindspots—one regarding our notion of punishment and the other our notion of moral responsibility. Regarding the first, if there is one insight into human behavior that the twentieth century should have firmly implanted, it is that punishment cannot be seen in merely physical terms, nor only from the perspective of the giver. Granted that capital offenses are on the decrease, that whipping and torture seem to be disappearing, as is the use of chains and other physical restraints, yet our ability if not willingness to inflict human anguish on one another does not seem similarly on the wane. The most effective forms of brain-washing deny any physical contact and the concept of relativism tells much about the psychological costs of even relative deprivation of tangible and intangible wants. Thus, when an individual because of his "disease" and its treatment is forbidden to have intercourse with fellow human beings, is confined until cured, is forced to undergo certain medical procedures for his own good, perhaps deprived forever of the right to have sexual relations and/or produce children, *then* it is difficult for that patient *not* to view what is happening to him as punishment. This does not mean that medicine is the latest form of twentieth-century torture, but merely that pain and suffering take many forms, and that the removal of a despicable inhumane procedure by current standards does not necessarily mean that its replacement will be all that beneficial. In part, the satisfaction in seeing the chains cast off by Pinel may have allowed us for far too long to neglect examining with what they had been replaced.

It is the second issue, that of responsibility, which requires more elaboration, for it is argued here that the medical model has had its greatest impact in the lifting of moral condemnation from the individual. While some skeptics note that while the individual is no longer condemned his disease still *is*, they do not go far enough. Most analysts have tried to make a distinction between illness and crime on the issue of personal responsibility.[8] The

criminal is thought to be responsible and therefore accountable (or punishable) for his act, while the sick person is not. While the distinction does exist, it seems to be more a quantitative one rather than a qualitative one, with moral judgments but a pinprick below the surface. For instance, while it is probably true that individuals are no longer directly condemned for being sick, it does seem that much of this condemnation is merely displaced. Though his immoral character is not demonstrated in his having a disease, it becomes evident in what he does about it. Without seeming ludicrous, if one listed the traits of people who break appointments, fail to follow treatment regimen, or even delay in seeking medical aid, one finds a long list of "personal flaws." Such people seem to be ever ignorant of the consequences of certain diseases, inaccurate as to symptomatology, unable to plan ahead or find time, burdened with shame, guilt, neurotic tendencies, haunted with traumatic medical experiences, or members of some lower status minority group—religious, ethnic, racial or socioeconomic. In short, they appear to be a sorely troubled if not disreputable group of people.

The argument need not rest at this level of analysis, for it is not clear that the issues of morality and individual responsibility have been fully banished from the etiological scene itself. At the same time as the label "illness" is being used to attribute "diminished responsibility" to a whole host of phenomena, the issue of "personal responsibility" seems to be re-emerging within medicine itself. Regardless of the truth and insights of the concepts of stress and the perspective of psychosomatics, whatever else they do, they bring man, *not* bacteria, to the center of the stage and lead thereby to a re-examination of the individual's role in his own demise, disability, and even recovery.

The case, however, need not be confined to professional concepts and their degree of acceptance, for we can look at the beliefs of the man in the street. As most surveys have reported, when an individual is asked what caused his diabetes, heart disease, upper respiratory infection, etc., we may be comforted by the scientific terminology if not the accuracy of his answers. Yet if we follow this questioning with the probe: "Why did you get X now?", or "Of all the people in your community, family, etc. who were exposed to X, why did you get . . . ?", then the rational

scientific veneer is pierced and the concern with personal and moral responsibility emerges quite strikingly. Indeed the issue "why me?" becomes of great concern and is generally expressed in quite moral terms of what they did wrong. It is possible to argue that here we are seeing a residue and that it will surely be different in the new generation. A recent experiment I conducted should cast some doubt on this. I asked a class of forty undergraduates, mostly aged seventeen, eighteen, and nineteen, to recall the last time they were sick, disabled, or hurt and then to record how they did or would have communicated this experience to a child under the age of five. The purpose of the assignment had nothing to do with the issue of responsibility and it is worth noting that there was no difference in the nature of the response between those who had or had not actually encountered children during their "illness." The responses speak for themselves.

The opening words of the sick, injured person to the query of the child were:
"I feel bad."
"I feel bad all over."
"I have a bad leg."
"I have a bad eye."
"I have a bad stomach ache."
"I have a bad pain."
"I have a bad cold."
The reply of the child was inevitable:
"What did you do wrong?"
The "ill person" in no case corrected the child's perspective but rather joined it at that level.
On bacteria:
"There are good germs and bad germs and sometimes the bad germs . . ."
On catching a cold:
"Well you know sometimes when your mother says, 'Wrap up or be careful or you'll catch a cold,' well I . . ."
On an eye sore:
"When you use certain kinds of things (mascara) near your eye you must be very careful and I was not . . ."
On a leg injury:
"You've always got to watch where you're going and I . . ."
Finally to the treatment phase:

On how drugs work:
  "You take this medicine and it attacks the bad parts . . . "
On how wounds are healed:
  "Within our body there are good forces and bad ones and when
  there is an injury, all the good ones . . . "
On pus:
  "That's the way the body gets rid of all its bad things . . . "
On general recovery:
  "If you are good and do all the things the doctor and your
  mother tell you, you will get better."

In short, on nearly every level, from getting sick to recovering,
a moral battle raged. This seems more than the mere anthro-
pomorphizing of a phenomenon to communicate it more simply
to children. Frankly, it seems hard to believe that the English
language is so poor that a *moral* rhetoric is needed to describe a
supposedly amoral phenomenon—illness.

In short, despite hopes to the contrary, the rhetoric of illness
by itself seems to provide no absolution from individual responsibility, accountability, and moral judgment.

THE MEDICALIZING OF SOCIETY

Perhaps it is possible that medicine is not devoid of a potential
for moralizing and social control. The first question becomes:
"What means are available to exercise it?" Freidson has stated a
major aspect of the process most succinctly: "The medical profession has first claim to jurisdiction over the label of illness and
anything to which it may be attached, irrespective of its capacity
to deal with it effectively."[9] For illustrative purposes this "attach-
ing" process may be categorized in four concrete ways: first,
through the expansion of what in life is deemed relevant to the
good practice of medicine; secondly, through the retention of
absolute control over certain technical procedures; thirdly,
through the retention of near absolute access to certain "taboo"
areas; and finally, through the expansion of what in medicine is
deemed relevant to the good practice of life.

1. *The expansion of what in life is deemed relevant to the good
practice of medicine.* The change of medicine's commitment

from a specific etiological model of disease to a multi-causal one and the greater acceptance of the concepts of comprehensive medicine, psychosomatics, etc. have enormously expanded that which is or can be relevant to the understanding, treatment, and even prevention of disease. Thus it is no longer necessary for the patient merely to divulge the symptoms of his body, but also the symptoms of daily living, his habits and his worries. Part of this is greatly facilitated in the "age of the computer," for what might be too embarrassing, or take too long, or be inefficient in a face-to-face encounter can now be asked and analyzed impersonally by the machine, and moreover be done before the patient ever sees the physician. With the advent of the computer a certain guarantee of privacy is necessarily lost, for while many physicians might have probed similar issues, the only place where the data were stored was in the mind of the doctor, and only rarely in the medical record. The computer, on the other hand, has a retrievable, transmittable, and almost inexhaustible memory.

It is not merely, however, the nature of the data needed to make more accurate diagnoses and treatments, but the perspective which accompanies it—a perspective which pushes the physician far beyond his office and the exercise of technical skills. To rehabilitate or at least alleviate many of the ravages of chronic disease, it has become increasingly necessary to intervene to change permanently the habits of a patient's lifetime—be they of working, sleeping, playing or eating. In prevention, the "extension into life" becomes even deeper, since the very idea of primary prevention means getting there *before* the disease process starts. The physician must not only seek out his clientele but once found must often convince them that they must do something *now* and perhaps at a time when the potential patient feels well or not especially troubled. If this in itself does not get the prevention-oriented physician involved in the workings of society, then the nature of "effective" mechanisms for intervention surely does, as illustrated by the statement of a physician trying to deal with health problems in the ghetto:

Any effort to improve the health of ghetto residents cannot be separated from equal and simultaneous efforts to remove the multi-

ple social, political and economic restraints currently imposed on inner city residents.[10]

Certain forms of social intervention and control emerge even when medicine comes to grips with some of its more traditional problems like heart disease and cancer. An increasing number of physicians feel that a change in diet may be the most effective deterrent to a number of cardio-vascular complications. They are, however, so perplexed as to how to get the general population to follow their recommendations that a leading article in a national magazine was entitled "To Save the Heart: Diet by Decree?"[11] It is obvious that there is an increasing pressure for more explicit sanctions against the tobacco companies and against high users to force both to desist. And what will be the implications of even stronger evidence which links age at parity, frequency of sexual intercourse, or the lack of male circumcision to the incidence of cervical cancer, can be left to our imagination!

2. *Through the retention of absolute control over certain technical procedures.* In particular this refers to skills which in certain jurisdictions are the very operational and legal definition of the practice of medicine—the right to do surgery and prescribe drugs. Both of these take medicine far beyond concern with ordinary organic disease.

In surgery this is seen in several different subspecialities. The plastic surgeon has at least participated in, if not helped perpetuate, certain aesthetic standards. What once was a practice confined to restoration has now expanded beyond the correction of certain traumatic or even congenital deformities to the creation of new physical properties, from size of nose to size of breast, as well as dealing with certain phenomena—wrinkles, sagging, etc.—formerly associated with the "natural" process of aging. Alterations in sexual and reproductive functioning have long been a medical concern. Yet today the frequency of hysterectomies seems not so highly correlated as one might think with the presence of organic disease. (What avenues the very possibility of sex change will open is anyone's guess.) Transplantations, despite their still relative infrequency, have had a tremendous effect on our very notions of death and dying. And at the other end of life's

continuum, since abortion is still essentially a surgical procedure, it is to the physician-surgeon that society is turning (and the physician-surgeon accepting) for criteria and guidelines.

In the exclusive right to prescribe and thus pronounce on and regulate drugs, the power of the physician is even more awesome. Forgetting for the moment our obsession with youth's "illegal" use of drugs, any observer can see, judging by sales alone, that the greatest increase in drug use over the last ten years has not been in the realm of treating any organic disease but in treating a large number of psychosocial states. Thus we have drugs for nearly every mood:

> to help us sleep or keep us awake
> to enhance our appetite or decrease it
> to tone down our energy level or to increase it
> to relieve our depression or stimulate our interest.

Recently the newspapers and more popular magazines, including some medical and scientific ones, have carried articles about drugs which may be effective peace pills or antiaggression tablets, enhance our memory, our perception, our intelligence, and our vision (spiritually or otherwise). This led to the easy prediction: "We will see new drugs, more targeted, more specific and more potent than anything we have . . . And many of these would be for people we would call healthy."[12] This statement, incidentally, was made not by a visionary science fiction writer but by a former commissioner of the United States Food and Drug Administration.

3. *Through the retention of near absolute access to certain "taboo" areas.* These "taboo" areas refer to medicine's almost exclusive license to examine and treat that most personal of individual possessions—the inner workings of our bodies and minds. My contention is that if anything can be shown in some way to affect the workings of the body and to a lesser extent the mind, then it can be labeled an "illness" itself or jurisdictionally "a medical problem." In a sheer statistical sense the import of this is especially great if we look at only four such problems—aging, drug addiction, alcoholism, and pregnancy. The first and last were once regarded as normal natural processes and the middle

two as human foibles and weaknesses. Now this has changed and to some extent medical specialities have emerged to meet these new needs. Numerically this expands medicine's involvement not only in a longer span of human existence, but it opens the possibility of medicine's services to millions if not billions of people. In the United States, at least, the implication of declaring alcoholism a disease (the possible import of a pending Supreme Court decision, as well as laws currently being introduced into several state legislatures), would reduce arrests in many jurisdictions by ten to fifty percent and transfer such "offenders," when "discovered," directly to a medical facility. It is pregnancy, however, which produces the most illuminating illustration. For, again in the United States, it was barely seventy years ago that virtually all births and the concomitants of birth occurred outside the hospital as well as outside medical supervision. I do not frankly have a documentary history, but as this medical claim was solidified, so too was medicine's claim to a whole host of related processes: not only to birth but to prenatal, postnatal, and pediatric care; not only to conception but to infertility; not only to the process of reproduction but to the process and problems of sexual activity itself; not only when life begins (in the issue of abortion) but whether it should be allowed to begin at all (e.g., in genetic counselling).

Partly through this foothold in the "taboo" areas and partly through the simple reduction of other resources, the physician is increasingly becoming the choice for help for many with personal and social problems. Thus a recent British study reported that within a five-year period there had been a notable increase (from 25 to 41 percent) in the proportion of the population willing to consult the physician with a personal problem.[13]

4. *Through the expansion of what in medicine is deemed relevant to the good practice of life.* Though in some ways this is the most powerful of all "the medicalizing of society" processes, the point can be made simply. Here we refer to the use of medical rhetoric and evidence in the arguments to advance any cause. For what Wootton attributed to psychiatry is no less true of medicine. To paraphrase her, today the prestige of *any* proposal is immensely enhanced, if not justified, when it is expressed in

the idiom of medical science. To say that many who use such labels are not professionals only begs the issue, for the public is only taking its cues from professionals who increasingly have been extending their expertise into the social sphere or have called for such an extension.[14] In politics one hears of the healthy or unhealthy economy or state. More concretely, the physical and mental health of American presidential candidates has been an issue in the last four elections and a recent book claimed to link faulty political decisions with faulty health.[15] For years we knew that the environment was unattractive, polluted, noisy, and in certain ways dying, but now we learn that its death may not be unrelated to our own demise. To end with a rather mundane if depressing example, there has always been a constant battle between school authorities and their charges on the basis of dress and such habits as smoking, but recently the issue was happily resolved for a local school administration when they declared that such restrictions were necessary for reasons of health.

THE POTENTIAL AND CONSEQUENCES OF MEDICAL CONTROL

The list of daily activities to which health can be related is ever growing and with the current operating perspective of medicine it seems infinitely expandable. The reasons are manifold. It is not merely that medicine has extended its jurisdiction to cover new problems,[16] or that doctors are professionally committed to finding disease,[17] or even that society keeps creating disease.[18] For if none of these obtained today, we would still find medicine exerting an enormous influence on society. The most powerful empirical stimulus for this is the realization of how much everyone has, or believes he has, something organically wrong with him, or, put more positively, how much can be done to make one feel, look, or function better.

The rates of "clinical entities" found on surveys or by periodic health examinations range upward from 50 to 80 percent of the population studied.[19] The Peckham study found that only 9 percent of their study group were free from clinical disorder. Moreover, they were even wary of this figure and noted in a footnote that, first, some of these 9 percent had subsequently died

of a heart attack, and, secondly, that the majority of those without disorder were under the age of five.[20] We used to rationalize that this high level of prevalence did not, however, translate itself into action since not only are rates of medical utilization not astonishingly high but they also have not gone up appreciably. Some recent studies, however, indicate that we may have been looking in the wrong place for this medical action. It has been noted in the United States and the United Kingdom that within a given twenty-four to thirty-six hour period, from 50 to 80 percent of the adult population have taken one or more "medical" drugs.[21]

The belief in the omnipresence of disorder is further enhanced by a reading of the scientific, pharmacological and medical literature, for there one finds a growing litany of indictments of "unhealthy" life activities. From sex to food, from aspirins to clothes, from driving your car to riding the surf, it seems that under certain conditions, or in combination with certain other substances or activities, or if done too much or too little, virtually anything can lead to certain medical problems. In short, I, at least, have finally been convinced that living is injurious to health. This remark is not meant as facetiously as it may sound. But rather every aspect of our daily life has in it elements of risk to health.

These facts take on particular importance not only when health becomes a paramount value in society, but also a phenomenon whose diagnosis and treatment has been restricted to a certain group. For this means that that group, perhaps unwittingly, is in a position to exercise great control and influence about what we should and should not do to attain that "paramount value."

Freidson in his recent book *Profession of Medicine* has very cogently analyzed why the expert in general and the medical expert in particular should be granted a certain autonomy in his researches, his diagnoses, and his recommended treatments.[22] On the other hand, when it comes to constraining or directing human behavior *because* of the data of researches, diagnoses, and treatments, a different situation obtains. For in these kinds of decisions it seems that too often the physician is guided not by his technical knowledge but by his values, or values latent in his very techniques.

Perhaps this issue of values can be clarified by reference to some not so randomly chosen medical problems: drug safety, genetic counseling, and automated multiphasic testing.

The issue of drug safety should seem straightforward, but both words in that phrase apparently can have some interesting flexibility—namely what is a drug and what is safe. During Prohibition in the United States alcohol was medically regarded as a drug and was often prescribed as a medicine. Yet in recent years, when the issue of dangerous substances and drugs has come up for discussion in medical circles, alcohol has been officially excluded from the debate. As for safety, many have applauded the AMA's judicious position in declaring the need for much more extensive, longitudinal research on marihuana, and their unwillingness to back legalization until much more data are in. This applause might be muted if the public read the 1970 Food and Drug Administration's "Blue Ribbon" Committee Report on the safety, quality, and efficacy of *all* medical drugs commercially and legally on the market since 1938.[23] Though appalled at the lack and quality of evidence of any sort, few recommendations were made for the withdrawal of drugs from the market. Moreover, there are no recorded cases of anyone dying from an overdose or of extensive adverse side effects from marihuana use; but the literature on the adverse effects of a whole host of "medical drugs" on the market today is legion.

It would seem that the value positions of those on both sides of the abortion issue need little documenting, but let us pause briefly at a field where "harder" scientists are at work—genetics. The issue of genetic counseling, or whether life should be allowed to begin at all, can only be an ever increasing one. As we learn more and more about congenital, inherited disorders or predispositions, and as the population size for whatever reason becomes more limited, then, inevitably, there will follow an attempt to improve the quality of the population which shall be produced. At a conference on the more limited concern of what to do when there is a documented probability of the offspring of certain unions being damaged, a position was taken that it was not necessary to pass laws or bar marriages that might produce such offspring. Recognizing the power and influence of medicine and the doctor, one of those present argued: "There is no reason why

sensible people could not be dissuaded from marrying if they know that one out of four of their children is likely to inherit a disease."[24] There are in this statement certain values on marriage and what it is or could be that, while they may be popular, are not necessarily shared by all. Thus, in addition to presenting the argument against marriage, it would seem that the doctor should—if he were to engage in the issue at all—present at the same time some of the other alternatives:

> Some "parents" could be willing to live with the risk that out of four children, three may turn out fine.
> Depending on the diagnostic procedures available they could take the risk and, if indications were negative, abort.
> If this risk were too great but the desire to bear children was there, and depending on the type of problem, artificial insemination might be a possibility.
> Barring all these and not wanting to take any risk, they could adopt children.
> Finally, there is the option of being married without having any children.

It is perhaps appropriate to end with a seemingly innocuous and technical advance in medicine, automatic multiphasic testing. It has been a procedure hailed as a boon to aid the doctor, if not replace him. While some have questioned the validity of all those test results and still others fear that it will lead to second-class medicine for already underprivileged populations, it is apparent that its major use to date and in the future may not be in promoting health or detecting disease to prevent it. Thus three large institutions are now or are planning to make use of this method, not to treat people, but to "deselect" them. The armed services use it to weed out the physically and mentally unfit, insurance companies to reject "uninsurables" and large industrial firms to point out "high risks." At a recent conference representatives of these same institutions were asked what responsibility they did, or would, recognize to those whom they have just informed that they have been "rejected" because of some physical or mental anomaly. They calmly and universally stated: none—neither to provide them with any appropriate aid nor even to insure that they get or be put in touch with any help.

CONCLUSION

C. S. Lewis warned us more than a quarter of a century ago that "man's power over Nature is really the power of some men over other men, with Nature as their instrument." The same could be said regarding man's power over health and illness, for the labels health and illness are remarkable "depoliticizers" of an issue. By locating the source and the treatment of problems in an individual, other levels of intervention are effectively closed. By the very acceptance of a specific behavior as an "illness," and the definition of illness as an undesirable state, the issue becomes not whether to deal with a particular problem, but *how* and *when*.[25] Thus the debate over homosexuality, drugs, or abortion becomes focused on the degree of sickness attached to the phenomenon in question or the extent of the health risk involved. And the more principled, more perplexing, or even moral issue, of *what* freedom should an individual have over his or her own body is shunted aside.

As stated in the very beginning, this "medicalizing of society" is as much a result of medicine's potential as it is of society's wish for medicine to use that potential. Why then has the focus been more on the medical potential than on the social desire? In part it is a function of space, but also of political expediency. For the time rapidly may be approaching when recourse to the populace's wishes may be impossible. Let me illustrate this with the statements of two medical scientists who, if they read this essay, would probably dismiss all my fears as groundless. The first was commenting on the ethical, moral, and legal procedures of the sex change operation:

> Physicians generally consider it unethical to destroy or alter tissue except in the presence of disease or deformity. The interference with a person's natural procreative function entails definite moral tenets, by which not only physicians but also the general public are influenced. The administration of physical harm as treatment for mental or behavioral problems—as corporal punishment, lobotomy for unmanageable psychotics and sterilization of criminals—is abhorrent in our society.[26]

Here he states, as almost an absolute condition of human nature, something which is at best a recent phenomenon. He seems to

forget that there were laws promulgating just such procedures through much of the twentieth century; that within the past few years, at least one Californian jurist ordered the sterilization of an unwed mother as a condition of probation; and that such procedures were done by Nazi scientists and physicians as part of a series of medical experiments. More recently, there is the misguided patriotism of the cancer researchers under contract to the United States Department of Defense who allowed their dying patients to be exposed to massive doses of radiation to analyze the psychological and physical results of simulated nuclear fallout. True, the experiments were stopped, but not until they had been going on for *eleven* years.

The second statement is by Francis Crick at a conference on the implications of certain genetic findings: "Some of the wild genetic proposals will never be adopted because the people will simply not stand for them."[27] Note where his emphasis is: on the people, not the scientist. In order, however, for the people to be concerned, to act and to protest, they must first be aware of what is going on. Yet in the very privatized nature of medical practice, plus the continued emphasis that certain expert judgments must be free from public scrutiny, there are certain processes which will prevent the public from ever knowing what has taken place and thus from doing something about it. Let me cite two examples.

> Recently, in a European country, I overheard the following conversation in a kidney dialysis unit. The chief was being questioned about whether or not there were self-help groups among his patients. "No," he almost shouted, "that is the last thing we want. Already the patients are sharing too much knowledge while they sit in the waiting room, thus making our task increasingly difficult. We are working now on a procedure to prevent them from ever meeting with one another."

The second example removes certain information even farther from public view.

> The issue of fluoridation in the United States has been for many years a hot political one. It was in the political arena because, in order to fluoridate local water supplies, the decision in many juris-

dictions had to be put to a popular referendum. And when it was, it was often defeated. A solution was found and a series of state laws were passed to make fluoridation a public health decision and to be treated, as all other public health decisions, by the medical officers best qualified to decide questions of such a technical, scientific, and medical nature.

Thus the issue at base here is the question of what factors are actually of a solely technical, scientific, and medical nature!

To return to our opening caution, this paper is not an attack on medicine so much as on a situation in which we find ourselves in the latter part of the twentieth century; for the medical area is the arena or the example *par excellence* of today's identity crisis— what is or will become of man. It is the battleground, not because there are visible threats and oppressors, but because they are almost invisible; not because the perspective, tools, and practitioners of medicine and the other helping professions are evil, but because they are not. It is so frightening because there are elements here of the banality of evil so uncomfortably written about by Hannah Arendt.[28] But here the danger is greater, for not only is the process masked as a technical, scientific, objective one, but one done for our own good. A few years ago a physician speculated on what, based on current knowledge, would be the composite picture of an individual with a low risk of developing atherosclerosis or coronary-artery disease. He would be

> an effeminate municipal worker or embalmer completely lacking in physical or mental alertness and without drive, ambition, or competitive spirit; who has never attempted to meet a deadline of any kind; a man with poor appetite, subsisting on fruits and vegetables laced with corn and whale oil, detesting tobacco, spurning ownership of radio, television, or motorcar, with full head of hair but scrawny and unathletic appearance, yet constantly straining his puny muscles by exercise. Low in income, blood pressure, blood sugar, uric acid and cholesterol, he has been taking nicotinic acid, pyridoxine, and long term anti-coagulant therapy ever since his prophylactic castration.[29]

Thus I fear with Freidson:

> A profession and a society which are so concerned with physical and functional well-being as to sacrifice civil liberty and moral integrity

must inevitably press for a "scientific" environment similar to that provided laying hens on progressive chicken farms—hens who produce eggs industriously and have no disease or other cares.[30]

Nor does it really matter if, instead of the above depressing picture, we were guaranteed six more inches in height, thirty more years of life, or drugs to expand our potentialities and potencies; we should still be able to ask, what do six more inches matter, in what kind of environment will the thirty additional years be spent, or who will decide what potentialities and potencies will be expanded and what curbed.

I must confess that given the road down which so much expertise has taken us, I am willing to live with some of the frustrations and even mistakes that will follow when the authority for many decisions becomes shared with those whose lives and activities are involved. For I am convinced that patients have so much to teach to their doctors, as do students their professors and children their parents.

NOTES

1. T. Szasz, *The Myth of Mental Illness* (New York: Harper & Row, 1961); and R. Leifer, *In the Name of Mental Health* (New York: Science House, 1969).
2. E.g., A. Toffler, *Future Shock* (New York: Random House, 1970); and P. E. Slater, *The Pursuit of Loneliness* (Boston: Beacon Press, 1970).
3. Such as B. Wootton, *Social Science and Social Pathology* (London: Allen and Unwin, 1959).
4. H. Sigerist, *Civilization and Disease* (New York: Cornell University Press, 1943).
5. M. Foucault, *Madness and Civilization* (New York: Pantheon, 1965); and Szasz, *Myth of Mental Illness*.
6. G. Rosen, *A History of Public Health* (New York: MC Publications, 1955); and G. Rosen, "The Evolution of Social Medicine," in *Handbook of Medical Sociology*, eds. H. E. Freeman, S. Levine, and L. G. Reeder (Englewood Cliffs, N. J.: Prentice-Hall, 1963), pp. 17–61.
7. Wootton, *Social Science and Social Pathology*, p. 206.
8. Two excellent discussions are found in V. Aubert and S. Messinger,

"The Criminal and the Sick," *Inquiry* 1 (1958): 137–60; and E. Freidson, *Profession of Medicine* (New York: Dodd-Mead, 1970), pp. 205–77.

9. Freidson, *Profession of Medicine*, p. 251.

10. J. C. Norman, "Medicine in the Ghetto," *New Engl. J. Med.* 281 (1969): 1271.

11. "To Save the Heart: Diet by Decree?" *Time Magazine*, January 10, 1968, p. 42.

12. J. L. Goddard, quoted in the *Boston Globe*, August 7, 1966.

13. K. Dunnell and A. Cartwright, *Medicine Takers, Prescribers and Hoarders* (Boston: Routledge and Kegan Paul, 1972).

14. E.g., S. Alinsky, "The Poor and the Powerful," in *Poverty and Mental Health*, Psychiat. Res. Rep. No. 21 of the American Psychiatric Assoc. (January 1967); and B. Wedge, "Psychiatry and International Affairs," *Science* 157 (1961): 281–85.

15. H. L'Etang, *The Pathology of Leadership* (New York: Hawthorne Books, 1970).

16. Szasz, *Myth of Mental Illness*; and Leifer, *In the Name of Mental Health*.

17. Freidson, *Profession of Medicine*; and T. Scheff, "Preferred Errors in Diagnoses," *Medical Care* 2 (1964): 166–72.

18. R. Dubos, *The Mirage of Health* (Garden City, N. Y.: Doubleday, 1959); and R. Dubos, *Mankind Adapting* (New Haven: Yale University Press, 1965).

19. E.g., the general summaries of J. W. Meigs, "Occupational Medicine," *New Engl. J. Med.* 264 (1961); 861–67; and G. S. Siegel, *Periodic Health Examinations—Abstracts from the Literature* (Washington, D.C.: Public Health Service Publication No. 1010, U.S. Government Printing Office, 1963).

20. I. H. Pearse and L. H. Crocker, *Biologists in Search of Material* (London: Faber and Faber, 1938); and I. H. Pearse and L. H. Crocker, *The Peckham Experiment* (London: Allen and Unwin, 1949).

21. Dunnell and Cartwright, *Medicine Taker, Prescribers and Hoarders*; and K. White, A. Andjelkovic, R. J. C. Pearson, J. H. Mabry, A. Ross, and O. K. Sagan, "International Comparisons of Medical Care Utilization," *New Engl. J. of Med.* 277 (1967): 516–22.

22. Freidson, *Profession of Medicine*.

23. *Drug Efficiency Study—Final Report to the Commissioner of Food and Drugs* (Washington, D.C.: Food and Drug Admin. Med. Nat. Res. Council, National Academy of Science 1969).

24. Reported in L. Eisenberg, "Genetics and the Survival of the Unfit," *Harper's Magazine* 232 (1966): 57.
25. This general case is argued more specifically in I. K. Zola, "Medicine, Morality, and Social Problems—Some Implications of the Label Mental Illness," paper presented at the American Ortho-Psychiatric Assoc., March 20–23, 1968.
26. D. H. Russell, "The Sex Conversion Controversy," *New Engl. J. Med.* 279 (1968): 536.
27. F. Crick, reported in *Time Magazine*, April 19, 1971.
28. H. Arendt, *Eichmann in Jerusalem—A Report on the Banality of Evil* (New York: Viking Press, 1963).
29. G. S. Myers, quoted in L. Lasagna, *Life, Death, and the Doctor* (New York: Alfred Knopf, 1968), pp. 215–16.
30. Freidson, *Profession of Medicine*, p. 354.

MARC RENAUD

ON THE STRUCTURAL CONSTRAINTS TO STATE INTERVENTION IN HEALTH

It is widely assumed that contemporary health problems may increasingly only be solved through the coercive legal powers and fiscal involvement of the state. The state is increasingly called into subsidizing part or the whole of the demand for medical care, into socializing certain costs of the production of care, and into issuing norms and standards for health care delivery, working conditions, environmental controls, drugs, food, and the like. The purpose of this paper is to explore the boundaries of state intervention in health. This essay attempts to identify the structural constraints which preselect the issues to which the state in capitalist societies is capable of responding, and consequently, which set the upper limits on what can be done by the state in order to improve the level of health in the population.

Beyond the most apparent and often nationally specific constraints, such as the existing institutional arrangements, the demands and pressures of interest groups, the electoral platforms of political parties, the national structure of political decision-making, and the inextricable problems of management and coordination embedded in a given health system, state interventions in the health field are bound everywhere in the capitalist world by less visible yet real constraints that are deeply rooted in the capitalist mode of production and that are largely above the volition of individual health-care workers, public officials, and the

Earlier drafts of this essay have benefited from the comments and criticisms of Robert R. Alford, Roger Friedland, Sander Kelman, James O'Connor, Louise Roy, and Julia Wrigley. Needless to say, the present version is entirely the author's own responsibility.

citizenry alike. It is argued here that capitalist industrial growth produces health needs that are treated by medicine in capitalist societies in such a way as to make the solutions to these needs compatible with the capitalist organization of the economy. The dominant engineering approach of contemporary scientific medicine equates healing and consumption, that is, in more general terms, health needs and the commodity form of their satisfaction, thus legitimating and facilitating capitalist economic growth despite its negative health consequences.

To the new diseases engendered by capitalist industrial growth, such as ischemic heart diseases, various cancers, and mental and nervous disorders, medicine has evolved an approach which is incapable of acting upon the social component of the etiology of diseases. Illness is reduced to being regarded as a natural process to be treated independently of its social causes by a vast array of experts utilizing the most complex technologies.

When the state intervenes to manage or prevent the crises provoked by some health-related problems, it cannot legitimately overcome the deeply embedded equation between healing and consumption: it can only further commodify health needs. In other words, the cause of the health-improvement ineffectiveness or of the class-biased characteristics of state intervention in the health field must not—although this might be critically important for a given public policy—fundamentally be searched for in the Machiavellian wills of some powerful individuals or groups under the control of some medical empire, but must rather be searched for in the institutionalized relationships between capitalism, health needs, medicine, and the state, which to an important extent predetermine the potential range of actions of individuals and groups.

HEALTH NEEDS IN ADVANCED CAPITALIST SOCIETIES

In order to identify the boundaries of state intervention in health, the existence of a paradox between "the enthusiasm associated with current developments and the reality of decreasing returns to health for rapidly increasing efforts" must first be recognized. Even though human beings in modern societies are

born, cured, checked up, and die in hospitals, surrounded by
impressive and costly technical apparatus and a complex division
of labor, even though it is widely believed that industrial populations owe their higher health standards to the development of
scientific medicine, and even though an unparalleled amount of
resources is invested in the health sector, there is an impressive
amount of evidence which shows that current health standards
derive less from new "discoveries" and technologies than from
the evolution of the environment within which human beings are
living, and that current scientific medicine produces more comfort than actual health. In this context, resource allocations to
health care seem to derive more from beliefs and traditions than
from evidence of their social utility. A brief overview of the
impact of medicine on infectious and chronic diseases will substantiate this assertion.

As Dubos has shown,[1] the great advances in health in the
eighteenth and nineteenth centuries were largely the result of
social reforms that alleviated some of the pollution, dirt, poor
housing and crowding, and malnutrition that had come from the
industrial revolution.[2] And although it is generally taken for
granted that the introduction of antibiotics and effective immunization campaigns were the key detemining factors in the
success of the fight against infectious diseases, Powles[3] and
McKeown[4] provide convincing evidence to the contrary. As
Powles writes:

> Whilst this may have been true in particular cases—for example,
> immunisation against diphtheria—their contribution to the total de-
> cline in mortality over the last two centuries has been a minor one.
> Most of the reduction had already occurred before they were intro-
> duced and there was only a slight downward inflection in an other-
> wise declining curve following their introduction.[5]

He then cites the research of Porter who

> recently plotted, for England and Wales, deaths in children under
> fifteen years attributed to scarlet fever, diphtheria, whooping cough,
> and measles in the period 1860–1965. Nearly 90 percent of the total
> decline in the death rate over this period had occurred before the
> introduction of antibiotics and what Porter refers to as "compulsory"

immunisation against diphtheria. . . . The provision of food, sanitary control and the regulation of births have been the three central factors.[6]

Similarly, McKeown argues that

The available evidence, scarce as it is, tends to show that medicine, to a significant extent, is not effective in its fight against chronic diseases. This does not mean that some individuals do not derive some benefit or cure from medicine but rather that, in the aggregate, medicine is far less effective than is generally taken for granted. Haggerty reviews some systematic mea-

until the second quarter of the twentieth century the decline of mortality from infections owed little to specific measures of preventing or treating disease in the individual. Mortality began to fall before identification of the causal organisms and, with the exception of smallpox whose contribution to the total reduction was small, long before the introduction of effective immunization or treatment.[7]

To be clear, immunization and antibiotics certainly are effective means to intervene in individuals and they have contributed to the almost total elimination of infectious diseases in advanced industrialized societies. The point is that resources have been invested for infectious diseases under the belief that immunization and antibiotics were the central causes of the diminution of mortality and morbidity from infections, while changes in the larger environment were, in fact, the prime causal factors.

The same point is valid for chronic diseases. Despite the constantly reinforced popular support from which it benefits, and the comparatively much higher amount of resources invested in it, the fight of scientific medicine against chronic diseases also seems only to have produced marginal gains in the improvement of health. For instance, in his *Effectiveness and Efficiency*, Cochrane calls for more controlled clinical trials to counter the uncritical beliefs in the virtues of modern medicine, pointing out that

environmental factors alone were important in improving vital statistics up to the end of the nineteenth century and that until the second quarter of this century therapy had very little effect on

morbidity and mortality. One should, therefore, forty years later, be delightfully surprised when any treatment at all is effective, and always assume that a treatment is ineffective unless there is evidence to the contrary.[8]

surements of the health-maintenance and health-improvement effectiveness of modern medicine.[9] These include a comparison of a costly versus a less costly treatment of myocardial infarction; comparisons of comprehensive medical care programs in the United States with the available care, albeit often fragmented, episodic, and uncoordinated as it is; the effects of the introduction of modern medical care in a primitive society versus the effects of no such introduction. He concludes:

> I need to make perfectly clear that I am well aware that we do have some data on the effectiveness of specific aspects of curative medicine—penicillin for pneumonia, antimicrobial treatment of meningitis, drug therapy for essential hypertension and a few other conditions that have been shown by controlled clinical trials to be positively affected by modern therapy. And I certainly do not wish to belittle the very important effects of our role as relievers of pain and distress. . . . [But] in sum, we can say that there is not much evidence that illness care (which is what most medical care consists of) reduces mortality and morbidity very much. When well organized, it can reduce utilization of expensive facilities such as hospitals and emergency rooms and can reduce other costs such as laboratory and pharmacy without any measurable difference in health status.[10]

Contrary to what is assumed by contemporary medicine, chronic diseases are to an important extent human beings' responses to environmental stimuli and insults. As Dubos says:

> Health and disease are the expressions of the relative degrees of success or failure experienced by man as he tries to respond adaptively to environmental challenges, and also to the inner demands created in him by traditions and aspirations. . . . Many, if not most, chronic disorders are the secondary and delayed consequences of adaptive responses that were useful at first, but are faulty in the long run. When evaluated over man's whole life span, homeostatic mechanisms are therefore less successful than commonly assumed.[11]

Specifically, the so-called diseases of civilization—ischemic heart disease, mental and nervous disorders, diabetes, and some forms of cancer—are not simply age-related degenerative processes but are, rather, consequences of changes in behavior associated with economic development, and of industrialization-induced changes in the natural environment. Powles suggests:

> Industrial populations owe their current health standards to a pattern of ecological relationships which serves to reduce their vulnerability to death from infection and to a lesser extent to the capabilities of clinical [both curative and preventive] medicine. Unfortunately this new way of life, because it is so far removed from that to which man is adapted by evolution, has produced its own disease burden. These diseases of maladaptation are, in many cases, increasing.[12]

In other words, our earlier evolution has "left us genetically unsuited for life in an industrialized society,"[13] and the costly and technologically specialized medical repair jobs, despite what appear to the layman as heroic efforts, largely seem incapable of coping with it.

Not only is medicine significantly incapable of dealing with the diseases generated by industrial development—except for some diseases and for symptomatic relief—but there is also evidence to show that medicine itself is producing its own disease burden. As Illich has documented, scientific medicine produces damage that outweighs its potential benefits, on what Illich terms clinical, social, and structural levels.[14] Modern professional health care systems are themselves intrinsically pathogenic because of their therapeutic side-effects, because of the deep dependency they create toward medical care, and because they "transform adaptive ability into consumer discipline"[15] so as to paralyze all healthy responses to suffering.

THE MEDICAL AND SOCIETAL RESPONSE

The issues then are the following: Why was the major thrust of the medical response to the new "diseases of civilization" to

create more and more costly technologies and facilities, given the absence of convincing evidence of benefit and given that there was evidence that changes in the larger environment played the critical role as the prime determining factor for the improvement of health? Why is it that countries invest between 5 and 10 percent of their gross national product in the health sector, while the very task of curing and preventing diseases is left unaccomplished, in that the most prevalent diseases—especially ischemic heart disease—are increasing and are killing people at younger ages? Why is it that the state supports medicine so heavily if indeed medicine does produce its own disease burden that outweighs its potential benefits?

The answers to these questions are obviously quite complex and they can only be highly tentative, but because they are so critical to understanding state intervention in health, answers must be provided, however incomplete and debatable they might be.

A familiar argument runs as follows. Human beings have always, throughout known history, culturally endowed certain persons with the authority to define health and illness and with the power to alleviate pain and distress, whether these persons be shamans, priests, or physicians, and whatever their objective effectiveness in curing diseases might be. Despite the proclaimed "rationality" and the idealized search for scientific efficiency in advanced capitalist societies, human beings still cannot escape from being frightened by death and sickness, thus building scientific medicine into a myth and investing the various therapeutic facilities with the appropriate rituals and value-content to celebrate this myth, independently of the costs involved and of their objective health-maintenance effectiveness.

Assuming this point of view to be valid, vital questions would remain unanswered: Why, despite its enormous costs, has modern scientific medicine so overshadowed other ways of dealing with sickness? And why have individuals been so isolated and atomized in their search for health? The key answer to these questions lies in the congruence between the dominant engineering approach within medicine and the larger capitalist environment.

Contemporary medical knowledge is rooted in the paradigm of the "specific etiology" of diseases, that is, diseases are assumed to have a specific cause to be analyzed in the body's cellular and biochemical systems. This paradigm developed out of the germ theory of disease of Pasteur and Koch. This theory contrasted with earlier theories based on the idea of human adaptation, which largely formed the foundation for the sanitary revolution in England in the mid-nineteenth century. While the works of Pasteur and Koch helped to prevent infectious diseases, by a paradoxical evolution of history, their paradigm gave support to the idea of specific therapies, from which arose the essentially curative orientation of current medical technologies toward specific illnesses rather than the sick person as a whole, and the belief that people can be made healthy by means of technological fixes, i.e., the engineering approach. This approach basically assumes, as McKeown says, that

> a living organism could be regarded as a machine which might be taken apart and reassembled if its structure and function were fully understood. In medicine the same concept led further to the belief that an understanding of disease processes and of the body's response to them would make it possible to intervene therapeutically, mainly by physical (surgical), chemical, or electrical methods. [16]

Because of the dominance of this paradigm, the idea was lost that diseases may be caused by a vast array of interlinked factors tied to the environment or, in other words, that diseases may be individually experienced problems of adaptation. The forgotten idea is what many, including Dreitzel[17] and Rossdale,[18] call the "ecological" approach to illness.

Examples of the pervasive dominance of this paradigm, however, abound. For instance, as Powles noted, it is significant that medical establishments were surprised that tobacco smoking actually harmed the lungs and caused cancer, and in some cases virtually opposed this idea. Similarly, it is because of this paradigm that medicine

> hesitates to call progressive health-compromising processes—such as arterial degeneration, rising blood pressure and tendency toward diabetes—"diseases" because they are associated with a way of life it feels bound to accept as "normal."[19]

It is also significant, to give yet one more instance, that the pathogenic effects of drugs are often underplayed.

This view of health and illness is congruent with the larger capitalist environment because it commodifies health needs and legitimates this commodification. It transforms the potentially explosive social problems that are diseases and death into discrete and isolable commodities that can be incorporated into the capitalist organization of the economy in the same way as any other commodity on the economic market. In an incredible *tour de force*, it succeeds in providing culturally valued solutions to problems largely created by economic growth, and even makes these solutions to a certain extent profitable for capital accumulation and thus for more economic growth. With scientific medicine, health care has grown into an industry which helps maintain the legitimacy of the social order, and which, in part, creates new sectors of production.

With such a paradigm, "society" is epistemologically eliminated as an important element in the etiology of disease, therefore impeding the growth of a consciousness of the harmfulness of economic growth. The engineering approach transforms the largely social determinants of morbidity and mortality into a value-loaded "rational" system of endogenous causes, thus obscuring the extent to which illness depends on socially determined ways of life and on the damaged natural environment—an enlightened consciousness of which would be potentially threatening to the social order.

In addition, with this paradigm, the treatment of disease does not, as in the past, involve the entire individual. Rather, the individual is isolated in the face of his or her sickness with the help of increasingly professionalized "experts," the physicians. This builds an extremely strong tie between the public and the physicians, whose healing powers, precisely because they are more apparent than real, reinforce the belief in the need for ever more expertise, i.e., in ever more consumption of "expert" services. As Illich has well expressed, "The patient is reduced to an object being repaired; he is no longer a subject being helped to heal."[20]

Finally, this paradigm stimulates the consumption by physicians of increasingly complex equipment and the prescription of

increasingly differentiated drugs. Members of the public, similarly, are stimulated to consume a myriad of specific products that supposedly will keep them healthy—such as vitamins, antidepressants, and ultraviolet lamps—in an endless search for health which, in the last analysis, profits those who capitalize on it more than it benefits the health of the public.

In brief, the isolation of the individual from his community, the isolation of the illness from the entire individual, the institutionalized expert solutions to health needs, and the endless consumption process that is unleashed, succeed in transforming health needs into commodities that are often provided profitably by economic interest, but which do not ameliorate the level of health in the population.

It remains an open question whether the "diseases of civilization" are tied to industrialization *per se* or whether they are linked to the specifically capitalist mode of economic growth. Sufficient, direct, and reliable evidence is not available. On the one hand, since these diseases derive from changes in behavior associated with economic development and from changes in the natural environment induced by industry, it is likely that they will be prevalent under industrialization in both its capitalist and socialist forms. On the other hand, however, since socialism, in theory if not in practice in the existing socialist societies, gives precedence to human needs rather than to capital accumulation, it is also likely that these diseases will be less prevalent with socialism. In any case, the key difference between the approaches to health in contemporary capitalist and socialist societies relates more to how medicine can cope with these diseases than to the sheer prevalence of the diseases. Under capitalism, because the engineering model of medicine institutionalizes a self-defeating dependence on economic growth to solve the problems associated with that growth, it is unlikely that viable solutions can be devised and put into effect to correct the conditions giving rise to these diseases. On the contrary, if we may believe certain reports,[21] there are signs that certain socialist societies are in a better position to implement a very different approach to health, illness, and medicine. If only because of the ideology behind them, all self-defined socialist health policies are more prone to be respon-

sive to issues such as the qualities of life at work, of food, and of the natural environment.

THE BOUNDARIES OF STATE INTERVENTION

When the state intervenes in the health sector, it has a quite wide range of potential actions, which vary from country to country according to differing institutional arrangements and class relationships, but, everywhere in the capitalist world, the range of state actions is limited by the fact that environmental health needs usually must be transformed into commodities to insure the survival of the capitalist organization of the economy. The state can only aggregate individual needs and social commodity exchanges into national budgets and plans, but it cannot reorganize the economy so that less illness is produced.

The state, in advanced capitalist societies, is the legitimate problem-solver, in that it cautiously manages crises and develops long-term avoidance strategies in an effort to fulfil two inherently contradictory functions: to sustain capital accumulation and to legitimize the social consequences of this accumulation. The state has the distinguishing feature of being the ultimate locus where contradictions have to be resolved and social tensions reduced for the social order to be maintained. Yet the state is not a neutral mechanism. It is not an arbiter between social classes, but an element in the class system itself. It must simultaneously maintain or improve the conditions for profitable capital accumulation, thus inevitably favoring those individuals who profit from this accumulation, while maintaining or improving the conditions for social harmony, i.e., it has to appear as a universal rather than a class-based state.[22]

In intervening in the health field, the state, then, must be responsive both to the economic requirements of the health industry and to the organized demands of the public. Schematically, there are two possibilities, the one in which a given public policy satisfies both needs and the one in which the demands and requirements do not coincide.

In the first instance the state can relatively easily intervene. This, for example, is the case with health insurance programs.

The considerable debates and political struggles which usually surround their enactment are only the public expression of the negotiating strategies of interest groups; they are the political rituals that create the beliefs and the expectations that help interest groups to maintain or improve their powers and privileges. To focus only on these debates and struggles obscures the extent to which much more sociologically important although less directly visible structural constraints and imperatives are at stake; these constraints and imperatives largely predetermine which issues get defined and who wins and who loses in a given confrontation.[23] On the other hand, when the economic requirements of the health industry as a whole and the demands of social movements do *not* coincide, the state is caught in a very precarious equilibrium, endlessly searching for legitimizing solutions to ever more exacerbated contradictions and social tensions. To substantiate these hypotheses, let us examine the internal dynamics of state intervention in health.

With the evolution of the medical engineering model toward increasingly specialized and differentiated products and services, the producers and providers of medical goods have gained considerable control over the health sector, to the extent that physicians have lost their entrepreneurial autonomy. Hospitals and drug and medical equipment manufacturers have increasingly become the heart of health-care delivery and, simultaneously, these organizations need ever more consumption of their services and goods in order to survive. They require ever more help from the state to maintain or improve the level of consumption, middle-income consumers having been priced out of the market.

With this evolution, various consumer groups and working-class movements filter out the health needs of the population and articulate demands for a more equal distribution of the culturally acclaimed blessings of modern medicine.

Because of pressures from above and from below, the state thus has to become responsive to issues of equity of access at a "reasonable" price to the consumer and at "reasonable" costs for its own fiscal capacity. This is what universal health insurance programs are all about: they maintain or improve the conditions for capital accumulation and they recreate social harmony by slightly

redistributing income. Paradoxically, they may be interpreted both as a "victory" for the working class, which "wins" easier access to medical services, and as a "victory" for the medical-care producers, because of the benefit that they get from increased consumption. That the use-value of such programs for satisfying the health needs of the population be nil is not at stake; what matters for the state is their exchange-value for popular support and their use-value for reproducing capitalism.

State intervention to maintain or extend the market for health goods or services automatically politicizes health-care delivery and imposes, in the short run, the necessity for some form of regulation—either through its own bureaucracy or through a delegation of state authority—the most important of which being the "planning" of the allocation of resources. Even though no precise norms of "what ought to be" can be agreed upon, the state has to find means to facilitate the geographical and financial access to physicians and to hospitals, and to limit the expensive competition among physicians, among hospitals, and among drug firms, but always with the objective of both satisfying the demand for care and maintaining the overall costs as low as possible.

But these two objectives are inherently contradictory because the demand for medical and hospital care is almost infinite or, more precisely, no country has ever experienced an end to it. It cannot be taken for granted that there is a limited quantity of diseases which, if appropriately reengineered by physicians, would result in a leveling off of the demand for care. The cause of this situation is not simply that people are hypochondriacs or that physicians only are income-maximizers utilizing hospital facilities as much as they can, but rather that the very medical care that people receive, as well as the very machinery used by physicians in hospitals, help to produce more comfort than actual health. Modern medicine does not deal with the environmental stimuli and insults which are the prime causes of disease; in fact, overmedicalization produces new diseases. In their search for health, people and physicians alike are thus led into constantly more consumption: more physician visits, more pills prescribed, more laboratory tests, and more surgery. And the state has to find

means to limit this increasingly expensive and partially health-damaging consumption.

Once the state subsidizes the consumption of medical care, it is thus caught in the internal contradictions of contemporary medical care. The problems of access inevitably lead to the problems of the costs, organization, and administration of health services.

Because an easier access to care brings about a higher demand for care and thus higher overall costs, or because of social movements clearly identifying and publicizing some health-damaging environmental conditions, the state may become concerned with issues related to the health-maintenance or health-improvement effectiveness of the health industry. This is where the structural constraints imposed by the economically determined equation between health needs and the commodity form of their satisfaction are more felt. The state is confronted by forces hopelessly outside of its reach.

The state cannot act against the alienation built into the work process in capitalist economies, even though the quality of the work process might be a prime determinant of diseases. As a Special Task Force to the Secretary of the Department of Health, Education, and Welfare recently noted in a report entitled *Work in America*:

> In an impressive fifteen-year study of aging, the strongest predictor of longevity was work satisfaction. The second best predictor was overall "happiness." . . . Other factors are undoubtedly important—diet, exercise, medical care, and genetic inheritance. But research findings suggest that these factors may account for only about 25 percent of the risk factors in heart disease, the major cause of death. That is, if cholesterol, blood pressure, smoking, glucose level, serum, uric acid, and so forth, were perfectly controlled, only about one-fourth of coronary heart disease could be controlled. Although research on this problem has not led to conclusive answers, it appears that work role, work conditions, and other social factors may contribute heavily to this "unexplained" 75 percent of risk factors. [24]

In its intervention, the state in capitalist societies cannot act directly or indirectly against the poor quality of work without threatening the accumulation process on which its own survival

in part depends. It cannot question the basic factor that makes work unhealthy: the fact that workers largely are only commodities utilized for maximum output, efficiency, and profit. It can only act on very limited, discrete, and easily identifiable working conditions.

The state cannot eliminate the artificial opulence created by capitalism; it can only publicize the needs for dieting and exercising, and for not smoking or drinking alcohol. It cannot stop automobile accidents; it can only coerce car manufacturers into engineering better cars and enforce the obligation to wear safety belts. It cannot eliminate the unhealthy comfort of our ways of life; it can only better analyze and regulate the production of drugs and food. It cannot eliminate the factors which account for the differential mortality and morbidity among social classes; it can only try to reduce the effects of some of them. It cannot suppress industries because people have too many accidents or because too many people die within them; it can only force workers to be more careful, or provide incentives for the elaboration of better protective devices or of better machines. It cannot eliminate the competitiveness which is stereotyped as successful even though it is a prime determinant of heart disease.

In brief, the state cannot reorganize the economy and correlated lifestyles so as to really provide solutions to health needs. At the limit, it can only try to compensate directly for the problems generated by capitalist economic growth, rather than indirectly through health services. If the state gets involved in this more direct form of compensation for health needs, it may intervene in three general directions that are compatible with capital accumulation in the economy as a whole, although they may not be congruent with accumulation in specific industries. They are discussed here in order of increasing difficulty of operationalization.

The first and easiest is to put the blame for bad health on the individual. And it can be done in many ways: by enforcing occupational health policies premised on the idea that most work-related health problems are due to workers' not being careful enough, not wearing the appropriate protective devices, and so on; by establishing publicity campaigns to encourage the public to

diet, to exercise, to relax, to quit smoking, and quit drinking alcohol; by legally enforcing the wearing of safety belts in automobiles; by evolving programs of immunization, screening, and follow-up. All these policies focus on individual at-risk behaviors and all have in common the imputation of responsibility on the individual. As McKinlay well describes it:

> [Individuals] are *either* doing something that they ought not to be doing, *or* they are not doing something that they ought to be doing. If only they would recognize their individual culpability and alter their behavior in some appropriate fashion, they would improve their health status or the likelihood of developing certain pathologies. . . . To use the upstream-downstream analogy, one could argue that people are blamed (and, in a sense, even punished) for not being able to swim after they, perhaps against their own volition, have been pushed into the river by the manufacturers of illness.[25]

State actions on at-risk behaviors are highly congruent with the bourgeois liberal vision of society according to which well-being derives from individual achievement, poverty from individual failure. They also do not challenge capital accumulation in other sectors of the economy, nor do they threaten the legitimacy of current medicine. On the contrary, such policies favor the development of whole new industries (e.g., diet foods, exercise equipment, differentiation of cigarette filters), and they, if successful, permit a more profitable utilization of a more healthy labor force. Moreover, the policies provide a highly valuable and strong argument to physicians when they cannot deal with, or explain, a given case. Rather than admit the weakness of the engineering model with which they work, they easily can blame the individual for his or her health problems.

A second avenue that the state can take concerns what McKinlay calls the "manufacturers of illness." This is a much more difficult and thus a less frequent type of intervention because it allegedly may, in the short run, threaten capital accumulation in some actually profitable sector of the economy. Moreover, because of the interests involved, it cannot come about without considerable input from working-class movements. The state can provide various incentives, e.g., socialization of certain costs,

charges for consumption, and establishment of long-term norms, in order to stimulate the development of antipollution devices, of better designed machines, of better occupational protective devices, of alternative chemical processes, and so on. Or, it can attempt to regulate certain industries, in particular food and drugs. But, in all cases, the state is self-defeatingly dependent upon economic growth to solve the problems associated with such growth. It is assumed here that new changes in technologies alone will improve the environment; yet, these new technologies might themselves bring new health problems that will again require new technological improvements, thus creating new problems.

A third possible avenue for the improvement of health through state actions is ultimately only possible in socialist societies, although some minor changes can realistically be expected within capitalist economies. It involves the implementation of an altogether different approach to health, disease, and medicine: in brief, the decommodification of health needs, leading to a more direct and intense preoccupation with the social conditions giving rise to disease. Specifically, it involves the development of a new medical knowledge based on what has been called an "ecological" approach, the elimination of the monopoly of the medical profession over the definition and cure of illnesses, the elimination of private property in skills, training, and credentials, and a reversal in the actual trends in the allocation of resources toward therapy and prevention, so that human beings can self-produce care of their bodies and minds, individually and socially.

Because the engineering approach within medicine simultaneously legitimates and reinforces capitalist economic growth and, needless to say, its wider organizational and cultural bases, it is intrinsically opposed to such policies. It is conceivable, however, that under certain social conditions, timid efforts could be made to partially implement a new, more preventive, and more community-oriented medicine, away from costly technologically specialized hospital-based medical practice. It is conceivable, for instance, that ambulatory care physicians, with more valued ancillary personnel, could become more aware of the need to teach their knowledge, of the global working and environmental char-

acteristics of the milieu where they practice, and of the entire personality of their patients, rather than only focus on their specific diseases in isolation from their community. The barriers that have to be overcome for the attainment of such a goal are very numerous, but not insuperable. The training of ambulatory care physicians has to be refocused, the resistances of already organized interest groups overcome, certain organizational incentives worked out, and so forth.

But state intervention within capitalist economies can only remain limited to the reorganization of a proportionally very small segment of the health sector, and even the health-maintenance or health-improvement effectiveness of such reforms can only be very limited. For larger forces—which are above the wills of physicians, public officials, and the public *alike*—impose the view that progress, in medicine and otherwise, is the sum total of ever more scientific expertise and technological advances, consumed by more and more individuals in ever greater quantity. Without a reversal in this view of progress and in its infrastructural determinants, it is unlikely that medicine and the social organization of health care will be fundamentally changed.

CONCLUSION

This paper has attempted to explore the general structural constraints which are imposed upon all states in capitalist societies in their problem-solving endeavors relative to health. The general argument has been that capitalist industrial growth both creates health needs and institutionalizes solutions to these needs that are compatible with capital accumulation. The key mechanism in this institutionalization is the medical engineering model which transforms health needs into commodities for a specific economic market. When the state intervenes, it is bound to act so as to further commodify health needs, thus favoring the unparalleled expansion of a sector of the civilian economy to the profit of those who capitalize on it, and thus further alienating individuals from control over their bodies and minds but without a significant improvement in the available indicators of the health status of the population.

It remains to be seen if the current efforts toward improving the quality of life in the natural environment, in working conditions, and in food, and toward implementing a new comprehensive social medicine, can succeed in ameliorating health. The deeply embedded and camouflaged logic of the capitalist social order in health predicts that partial successes can be obtained only at the price of considerable struggle. The conditions of success are embedded in the historically and nationally specific evolution of class relationships and they largely can only be understood in relation to specific political and economic conjunctures.[26]

NOTES

1. R. Dubos, *Mirage of Health: Utopias, Progress and Biological Change* (New York: Doubleday, 1959).
2. R. J. Haggerty, "The Boundaries of Health Care," *The Pharos of Alpha Omega Alpha* 35, no. 3 (1972): 106–11.
3. J. Powles, "On the Limitations of Modern Medicine," *Science, Medicine, and Man* 1, no. 1 (1973): 1–30.
4. T. McKeown, "An Historical Appraisal of the Medical Task," in *Medical History and Medical Care: A Symposium of Perspectives*, ed. T. McKeown and G. McLachlan (New York: Oxford University Press, 1971), pp. 29–55.
5. Powles, "On the Limitations of Modern Medicine," p. 6.
6. R. R. Porter, "The Contribution of the Biological and Medical Sciences to Human Welfare," in *Presidential Addresses of the British Association for the Advancement of Science, Swansea Meeting, 1971*, p. 95 (quoted in Powles, "On the Limitations of Modern Medicine").
7. McKeown, "Historical Appraisal of the Medical Task," p. 32.
8. A. L. Cochrane, *Effectiveness and Efficiency: Random Reflections on Health Services* (London: Nuffield Provincial Hospitals Trust, 1972), p. 8.
9. Haggerty, "Boundaries of Health Care."
10. Ibid., p. 107.
11. R. Dubos, "The Biology of Civilization—With Emphasis on Perinatal Influences," in *The Impact of Civilization on the Biology of Man*, ed. S. V. Boyden, Proceedings of the Symposium of the Australian Academy of Sciences, Canberra, 1968 (Toronto: University of Toronto Press, 1971), pp. 220–21.
12. Powles, "On the Limitations of Modern Medicine," p. 12.

13. G. Rose, "Epidemiology of Ischaemic Heart Disease," *Br. J. Hosp. Med.* 7, no. 3 (1972): 285–88 (quoted in Powles, "On the Limitations of Modern Medicine").

14. I. Illich, *Medical Nemesis: The Expropriation of Health* (Cuernavaca, Mexico; Center for Intercultural Documentation, 1974).

15. Ibid., p. 34.

16. McKeown, "Historical Appraisal of the Medical Task," p. 29.

17. *The Social Organization of Health*, ed. H. P. Dreitzel (New York: Macmillan, 1971).

18. M. Rossdale, "Health in a Sick Society," *New Left Review* 34 (1965): 82–90.

19. Powles, "On the Limitations of Modern Medicine," p. 14.

20. Illich, *Medical Nemesis*, p. 84.

21. See, for example, J. S. Horn, *Away with All Pests: An English Surgeon in People's China* (New York: Monthly Review Press, 1969); A. Peyrefitte, *Quand la Chine s'éveillera* . . . (Paris: Librairie Arthème Fayard, 1973); and M.-A. Macciocchi, *De la Chine* (Paris: Editions du Seuil, 1974).

22. C. Offe, "Political Authority and Class Structure: An Analysis of Late Capitalist Societies," *International Journal of Sociology* 2, no. 1 (1972): 73–108; C. Offe, "Advanced Capitalism and the Welfare State," *Politics and Society* 2, no. 4 (1972): 479–88; J. O'Connor, *The Fiscal Crisis of the State* (New York: St. Martin's Press, 1973); A. Wolfe, "New Directions in the Marxist Theory of Politics," *Politics and Society* 4, no. 2 (1974); 131–59.

23. R. R. Alford, "Towards a Critical Sociology of Political Power: Political Sociology Versus Political Economy in the Theory of the State," paper delivered at the meeting of the American Sociological Association, New York, August 1973.

24. Special Task Force to the Secretary of Health, Education, and Welfare, *Work in America* (Cambridge, Mass.: MIT Press, 1973), pp. 77–79.

25. J. B. McKinlay, "A Case for Refocussing Upstream: The Political Economy of Illness," unpublished paper (Boston University, 1974), p. 18.

26. M. Renaud, "The Political Economy of the Quebec State Interventions in Health: Reform or Revolution?" (Ph.D. diss., Madison, Wisconsin).

PART 2

MEDICINE AND WOMEN: A CASE STUDY IN SOCIAL CONTROL

BARBARA EHRENREICH AND DEIRDRE ENGLISH

THE "SICK" WOMEN OF THE UPPER CLASSES

The affluent woman of the late nineteenth century normally spent a hushed and peaceful life indoors, sewing, sketching, reading romances, planning menus, and supervising servants and children. Her clothes, a sort of portable prison of tight corsets and long skirts, prevented activity any more vigorous than a Sunday stroll. Society agreed that she was frail and sickly. Her delicate nervous system had to be shielded as carefully as her body, for the slightest shock could send her reeling off to bed. Elizabeth Barrett Browning, for example, although she was an extraordinarily productive woman, spent six years in bed following her brother's death in a sailboat accident.

But not even the most sheltered woman lived in a vacuum. Just outside the suffocating world of the parlor and the boudoir lay a world of industrial horror. This was the period of America's industrial revolution, a revolution based on the ruthless exploitation of working people. Women, and children as young as six, worked fourteen-hour days in factories and sweatshops for sub-subsistence wages. Labor struggles were violent, bordering, at times, on civil wars. For businessmen, too, survival was a bitter struggle: you squeezed what you could out of the workers, screwed the competition, and the devil take the hindmost. Fortunes were made and destroyed overnight, and with them rode the fates of thousands of smaller businessmen.

The genteel lady of leisure was not just an anomaly in an otherwise dog-eat-dog world. She was as much a product of that world as her husband or his employees. It was the wealth extracted in that harsh outside world that enabled a man to afford a

totally leisured wife. She was the social ornament that proved a man's success: her idleness, her delicacy, her childlike ignorance of "reality" gave a man the "class" that money alone could not provide. And it was the very harshness of the outside world that led men to see the home as a refuge—"a sacred place, a vestal temple," a "tent pitch'd in a world not right," presided over by a gentle, ethereal wife. Among the affluent classes, the worlds of men and women drifted farther and farther apart, with divergent standards of decorum, of health, of morality itself.

There were exceptional women in the upper classes—women who rebelled against the life of enforced leisure, the limitations on meaningful work—and it is these exceptional women who usually are remembered in history books. Many became women's rights activists or social reformers. A brave few struggled to make their way in the professions. And toward the end of the nineteenth century a growing number were demanding, and getting, college educations. But the majority of upper- and upper-middle-class women had little chance to make independent lives for themselves; they were financially at the mercy of husbands or fathers. They had to accept their roles—outwardly at least—and remain dutifully housebound, white-gloved, and ornamental. Of course, only a small minority of urban women could afford a life of total leisure, but a great many more women in the middle class aspired to it and did their best to live like "ladies."

THE CULT OF FEMALE INVALIDISM

The boredom and confinement of affluent women fostered a morbid cult of hypochondria—"female invalidism"—that began in the mid-nineteenth century and did not completely fade until the late 1910s. Sickness pervaded upper- and upper-middle-class female culture. Health spas and female specialists sprang up everywhere and became part of the regular circuit of fashionable women. And in the 1850s a steady stream of popular home readers by doctors appeared, all on the subject of female health. Literature aimed at female readers lingered on the romantic pathos of illness and death; popular women's magazines featured such stories as "The Grave of My Friend" and "Song of Dying."

Paleness and lassitude (along with filmy white gowns) came into vogue. It was acceptable, even fashionable, to retire to bed with "sick headaches," "nerves," and a host of other mysterious ailments.

In response, feminist writers and female doctors expressed their dismay at the chronic invalidism of affluent women. Dr. Mary Putnam Jacobi, an outstanding woman doctor of the late nineteenth century, wrote in 1895:

> It is considered natural and almost laudable to break down under all conceivable varieties of strain—a winter dissipation, a houseful of servants, a quarrel with a female friend, not to speak of more legitimate reasons. . . . Women who expect to go to bed every menstrual period expect to collapse if by chance they find themselves on their feet for a few hours during such a crisis. Constantly considering their nerves, urged to consider them by well-intentioned but short-sighted advisors, they pretty soon become nothing but a bundle of nerves.

Charlotte Perkins Gilman, the feminist writer and economist, concluded bitterly that American men "have bred a race of women weak enough to be handed about like invalids; or mentally weak enough to pretend they are—and to like it."

It is impossible to tell, in retrospect, how sick upper-middle-class women really were. Life expectancies for women were slightly higher than for men though the difference was nowhere near as great as it is today.

It is true, however, that women—*all* women—faced certain risks that men did not share, or share to the same degree. First were the risks associated with childbearing, which were all the greater in an age of primitive obstetrical technique when little was known about the importance of prenatal nutrition. In 1915 (the first year for which national figures are available) 61 women died for every 10,000 live babies born, compared to 2 for every 10,000 today, and the maternal mortality rates were doubtless higher in the nineteenth century. Without adequate, and usually without any, means of contraception, a married woman could expect to face the risk of childbirth repeatedly through her fertile years. After each childbirth a woman might suffer any number of

gynecological complications, such as a prolapsed (slipped) uterus or irreparable pelvic tear, which would stay with her for the rest of her life.

Another special risk to women came with tuberculosis, the "white plague." In the mid-nineteenth century, TB raged at epidemic proportions, and it continued to be a major threat until well into the twentieth century. Everyone was affected, but women, especially young women, were particularly vulnerable, often dying at rates twice as high as those of men of their age group. For every hundred women aged twenty in 1865, more than five would be dead from TB by the age of thirty, and more than eight would be dead by the age of fifty. (It is now believed that hormonal changes associated with puberty and childbearing accounted for the greater vulnerability of young women to TB.)

The dangers of childbearing, and of TB, must have shadowed women's lives in a way that we no longer know. But these dangers cannot explain the cultural phenomenon of "female invalidism" which, unlike TB and maternal mortality, was confined to women of a particular social class. The most important legitimization of this fashion came not from the actual dangers faced by women but from the medical profession.

The medical view of women's health not only acknowledged the specific risks associated with reproductivity; it went much farther: it identified *all* female functions as *inherently* sick. Puberty was seen as a "crisis," throwing the entire female organism into turmoil. Menstruation—or the lack of it—was regarded as pathological throughout a woman's life. Dr. W. C. Taylor, in his book *A Physician's Counsels to Woman in Health and Disease* (1871), gave a warning typical of those found in popular health books of the time:

> We cannot too emphatically urge the importance of regarding these monthly returns as periods of ill health, as days when the ordinary occupations are to be suspended or modified. . . . Long walks, dancing, shopping, riding and parties should be avoided at this time of month invariably and under all circumstances. . . . Another reason why every woman should look upon herself as an invalid once a month, is that the monthly flow aggravates any existing affection of the womb and readily rekindles the expiring flames of disease.

Similarly, a pregnant woman was "indisposed," and doctors campaigned against the practice of midwifery on the grounds that pregnancy was a disease and demanded the care of a doctor. Menopause was the final, incurable ill, the "death of the woman in the woman."

Women's greater susceptibility to TB was seen as proof of the inherent defectiveness of female physiology. Dr. Azell Ames wrote in 1875: "It being beyond doubt that consumption . . . is itself produced by the failure of the [menstrual] function in the forming girls . . . one has been the parent of the other with interchangeable priority." Actually, as we know today, it is true that consumption may *result* in suspension of the menses. But at that time consumption was blamed on woman's nature and on her reproductive system. When men were consumptive, doctors sought some environmental factor, such as overexposure, to explain the disease. But in popular imagery, consumption was always effeminate: novels of the time usually featured as male consumptives only such "effete" types as poets, artists, and other men "incompetent" for serious masculine pursuits.

The association of TB with innate feminine weakness was strengthened by the fact that TB is accompanied by an erratic emotional pattern in which a person may behave sometimes frenetically, sometimes morbidly. The behavior characteristic for the disease fit expectations about woman's personality, and the look of the disease suited—and perhaps helped to create—the prevailing standards of female beauty. The female consumptive did not lose her feminine identity, she embodied it: the bright eyes, translucent skin, and red lips were only an extreme of traditional female beauty. A romantic myth rose up around the figure of the female consumptive and was reflected in portraiture and literature; for example, in the sweet and tragic character of Beth, in *Little Women*. Not only were women seen as sickly—sickness was seen as feminine.

The doctors' view of women as innately sick did not, of course, *make* them sick, or delicate, or idle. But it did provide a powerful rationale against allowing women to act in any other way. Medical arguments were used to explain why women should be barred from medical school (they would faint in anatomy lectures), from

higher education altogether, and from voting. For example, a Massachusetts legislator proclaimed: "Grant suffrage to women, and you will have to build insane asylums in every county, and establish a divorce court in every town. Women are too nervous and hysterical to enter into politics." Medical arguments seemed to take the malice out of sexual oppression: when you prevented a woman from doing anything active or interesting, you were only doing this for her own good.

THE DOCTORS' STAKE IN WOMEN'S ILLNESS

The myth of female frailty, and the very real cult of female hypochondria that seemed to support the myth, played directly to the financial interests of the medical profession. In the late nineteenth and early twentieth centuries, the "regular" AMA doctors (members of the American Medical Association—the intellectual ancestors of today's doctors) still had no legal monopoly over medical practice and no legal control over the number of people who called themselves "doctors." Competition from lay healers of both sexes, and from what the AMA saw as an excess of formally trained male physicians, had the doctors running scared. A good part of the competition was female: women lay healers and midwives dominated the urban ghettos and the countryside in many areas; suffragists were beating on the doors of the medical schools.

For the doctors, the myth of female frailty thus served two purposes. It helped them to disqualify women as healers, and, of course, it made women highly qualified as patients. In 1900 there were 173 doctors engaged in primary patient care per 100,000 population, compared to 50 per 100,000 today. So, it was in the interests of doctors to cultivate the illnesses of their patients with frequent home visits and drawn-out "treatments." A few dozen well-heeled lady customers were all that a doctor needed for a successful urban practice. Women—at least, women whose husbands could pay the bills—became a natural "client caste" to the developing medical profession.

In many ways, the upper-middle-class woman was the ideal patient: her illnesses—and her husband's bank account—seemed almost inexhaustible. Furthermore, she was usually submissive

and obedient to the "doctor's orders." The famous Philadelphia doctor S. Weir Mitchell expressed his profession's deep appreciation of the female invalid in 1888:

> With all her weakness, her unstable emotionality, her tendency to morally warp when long nervously ill, she is then far easier to deal with, far more amenable to reason, far more sure to be comfortable as a patient, than the man who is relatively in a like position. The reasons for this are too obvious to delay me here, and physicians accustomed to deal with both sexes as sick people will be apt to justify my position.

In Mitchell's mind women were not only easier to relate to, but sickness was the very key to femininity: "The man who does not know sick women does not know women."

Some women were quick to place at least some of the blame for female invalidism on the doctors' interests. Dr. Elizabeth Garrett Anderson, an American woman doctor, argued that the extent of female invalidism was much exaggerated by male doctors and that women's natural functions were not really all that debilitating. In the working classes, she observed, work went on during menstruation "without intermission, and, as a rule, without ill effects." (Of course, working-class women could not have afforded the costly medical attention required for female invalidism.) Mary Livermore, a women's suffrage worker, spoke against "the monstrous assumption that woman is a natural invalid," and denounced "the unclean army of 'gynecologists' who seem desirous to convince women that they possess but one set of organs—and that these are always diseased." And Dr. Mary Putnam Jacobi put the matter most forcefully when she wrote in 1895, "I think, finally, it is in the increased attention paid to women, and especially in their new function as lucrative patients, scarcely imagined a hundred years ago, that we find explanation for much of the ill-health among women, freshly discovered today."

THE "SCIENTIFIC" EXPLANATION OF FEMALE FRAILTY

As a businessman, the doctor had a direct interest in a social role for women that encouraged them to be sick; as a doctor, he

had an obligation to find the causes of female complaints. The result was that as a "scientist," he ended up proposing medical theories that were actually justifications of women's social role.

This was easy enough to do at the time: no one had a very clear idea of human physiology. American medical education, even at the best schools, put few constraints on the doctors' imaginations, offering only a scant introduction to what was known of physiology and anatomy and no training in rigorous scientific method. So doctors had considerable intellectual license to devise whatever theories seemed socially appropriate.

Generally, they traced female disorders either to women's inherent "defectiveness" or to any sort of activity beyond the mildest "feminine" pursuits—especially sexual, athletic, and mental activity. Thus promiscuity, dancing in hot rooms, and subjection to an overly romantic husband were given as the origins of illness, along with too much reading, too much seriousness or ambition, and worrying.

The underlying medical theory of women's weakness rested on what doctors considered the most basic physiological law: "conservation of energy." According to the first postulate of this theory, each human body contained a set quantity of energy that was directed variously from one organ or function to another. This meant that you could develop one organ or ability only at the expense of others, drawing energy away from the parts not being developed. In particular, the sexual organs competed with the other organs for the body's fixed supply of vital energy. The second postulate of this theory—that reproductivity was central to a woman's biological life—made this competition highly unequal, with the reproductive organs in almost total command of the whole woman.

The implications of the "conservation of energy" theory for male and female roles are important. Let's consider them.

Curiously, from a scientific perspective, *men* didn't jeopardize their reproductivity by engaging in intellectual pursuits. On the contrary, since the mission of upper- and upper-middle-class men was to be doers, not breeders, they had to be careful not to let sex drain energy away from their "higher functions." Doctors warned men not to "spend their seed" (i.e., the essence of their energy)

recklessly, but to conserve themselves for the "civilizing endeavors" they were embarked upon. College youths were jealously segregated from women—except on rare sexual sprees in town—and virginity was often prized in men as well as women. Debilitated sperm would result from too much "indulgence," and this in turn could produce "runts," feeble infants, and girls.

On the other hand, because reproduction was woman's grand purpose in life, doctors agreed that women ought to concentrate their physical energy internally, toward the womb. All other activity should be slowed down or stopped during the peak periods of sexual energy use. At the onset of menstruation, women were told to take a great deal of bed rest in order to help focus their strength on regulating their periods—though this might take years. The more time a pregnant woman spent lying down quietly, the better. At menopause, women were often put to bed again.

Doctors and educators were quick to draw the obvious conclusion that, for women, higher education could be physically dangerous. Too much development of the brain, they counseled, would atrophy the uterus. Reproductive development was totally antagonistic to mental development. In a work entitled *Concerning the Physiological and Intellectual Weakness of Women*, the German scientist P. Moebius wrote:

> If we wish woman to fulfill the task of motherhood fully she cannot possess a masculine brain. If the feminine abilities were developed to the same degree as those of the male, her maternal organs would suffer and we should have before us a repulsive and useless hybrid.

In the United States this thesis was set forth most cogently by Dr. Edward Clarke of Harvard College. He warned, in his influential book *Sex in Education* (1873), that higher education was *already* destroying the reproductive abilities of American women.

Even if a woman should choose to devote herself to intellectual or other "unwomanly" pursuits, she could hardly hope to escape the domination of her uterus and ovaries. In *The Diseases of Woman* (1849), Dr. F. Hollick wrote: "The Uterus, it must be remembered, is the *controlling* organ in the female body, being the most excitable of all, and so intimately connected, by the

ramifications of its numerous nerves, with every other part." To other medical theorists, it was the ovaries that occupied center stage. This passage, written in 1870 by Dr. W. W. Bliss, is, if somewhat overwrought, nonetheless typical:

> Accepting, then, these views of the gigantic power and influence of the ovaries over the whole animal economy of woman,—that they are the most powerful agents in all the commotions of her system; that on them rest her intellectual standing in society, her physical perfection, and all that lends beauty to those fine and delicate contours which are constant objects of admiration, all that is great, noble and beautiful, all that is voluptuous, tender, and endearing; that her fidelity, her devotedness, her perpetual vigilance, forecast, and all those qualities of mind and disposition which inspire respect and love and fit her as the safest counsellor and friend of man, spring from the ovaries,—*what must be their influence and power over the great vocation of woman and the august purposes of her existence when these organs have become compromised through disease!* Can the record of woman's mission on earth be otherwise than filled with tales of sorrow, sufferings, and manifold infirmities, all through the influence of these important organs?

This was not mere textbook rhetoric. In their actual medical practices, doctors found uterine and ovarian "disorders" behind almost every female complaint, from headaches to sore throats and indigestion. Curvature of the spine, bad posture, or pains anywhere in the lower half of the body could be the result of "displacement" of the womb, and one doctor ingeniously explained how constipation results from the pressure of the uterus on the rectum. Dr. M. E. Dirix wrote in 1869:

> Thus, women are treated for diseases of the stomach, liver, kidneys, heart, lungs, etc.; yet, in most instances, these diseases will be found, on due investigation, to be, in reality, no diseases at all, but merely the sympathetic reactions or the symptoms of one disease, namely, a disease of the womb.

THE PSYCHOLOGY OF THE OVARY

If the uterus and ovaries could dominate woman's entire body, it was only a short step to the ovarian takeover of woman's entire

personality. The basic idea, in the nineteenth century, was that female psychology functioned merely as an extension of female reproductivity, and that woman's nature was determined solely by her reproductive functions. The typical medical view was that "The ovaries . . . give to woman all her characteristics of body and mind. . . ." And Dr. Bliss remarked, somewhat spitefully, "The influence of the ovaries over the mind is displayed in woman's artfulness and dissimulation." According to this "psychology of the ovary," all woman's "natural" characteristics were directed from the ovaries, and any abnormalities—from irritability to insanity—could be attributed to some ovarian disease. As one doctor wrote, "All the various and manifold derangements of the reproductive system, peculiar to females, add to the causes of insanity." Conversely, actual physical reproductive problems and diseases, including cancer, could be traced to bad habits and attitudes.

Masturbation was seen as a particularly vicious character defect that led to physical damage, and although this was believed to be true for both men and women, doctors seemed more alarmed by female masturbation. They warned that "The Vice" could lead to menstrual dysfunction, uterine disease, and lesions on the genitals. Masturbation was one form of "hypersexuality," which was said to lead to consumption; in turn, consumption might result in hypersexuality. The association between "hypersexuality" and TB was easily "demonstrated" by pointing to the high rates of TB among prostitutes. All this fueled the notion that "sexual disorders" led to disease, and conversely, that disease lay behind women's sexual desires.

The medical model of female nature, embodied in the "psychology of the ovary," drew a rigid distinction between reproductivity and sexuality. Women were urged by the health books and the doctors to indulge in deep preoccupation with themselves as "The Sex"; they were to devote themselves to developing their reproductive powers, their maternal instincts, their "femininity." Yet they were told that they had no "natural" sexual feelings whatsoever. They were believed to be completely governed by their ovaries and uteruses, but to be repelled by the sex act itself. In fact, sexual feelings were seen as unwomanly, pathological,

and possibly detrimental to the supreme function of reproduction. (Men, on the other hand, *were* believed to have sexual feelings, and many doctors went so far as to condone prostitution on the grounds that the lust of upper-middle-class males should have some outlet other than their delicate wives.)

The doctors themselves never seemed entirely convinced of this view of female nature. While they denied the existence of female sexuality as vigorously as any other men of their times, they were always on the lookout for it. Medically, this vigilance was justified by the idea that female sexuality could only be pathological. So it was only natural for some doctors to test for it by stroking the breasts or the clitoris. But under the stern disapproval, there always lurked the age-old fear of and fascination with woman's "insatiable lust" that, once awakened, might be totally uncontrollable. In 1853, when he was only twenty-five years old, the British physician Robert Brudenell Carter wrote (in a work entitled *On the Pathology and Treatment of Hysteria*):

> No one who has realized the amount of moral evil wrought in girls . . . whose prurient desires have been increased by Indian hemp and partially gratified by medical manipulations, can deny that remedy is worse than disease. I have . . . seen young unmarried women, of the middle class of society, reduced by the constant use of the speculum to the mental and moral condition of prostitutes; seeking to give themselves the same indulgence by the practice of solitary vice; and asking every medical practitioner . . . to institute an examination of the sexual organs.

(Did Dr. Carter's patients actually smoke "Indian hemp" or beg for internal examinations? Unfortunately, we have no other authority on the subject than Dr. Carter himself.)

MEDICAL TREATMENTS

Uninformed by anything that we would recognize today as a scientific description of the way human bodies work, the actual practice of medicine at the turn of the century was largely a matter of guesswork, consisting mainly of ancient remedies and occasional daring experiments. Not until 1912, according to one medical estimate, did the average patient, seeking help from the

average American doctor, have more than a fifty-fifty chance of benefiting from the encounter. In fact, the average patient ran a significant risk of actually getting worse as a result: bleeding, violent purges, heavy doses of mercury-based drugs, and even opium were standard therapeutic approaches throughout the nineteenth century, for male as well as female patients. Even well into the twentieth century, there was little that we would recognize as modern medical technology. Surgery was still a highly risky enterprise; there were no antibiotics or other "wonder drugs"; and little was understood, medically, of the relationship between nutrition and health or of the role of hormones in regulating physiological processes.

Every patient suffered from this kind of hit-or-miss treatment, but some of the treatments applied to women now seem particularly useless and bizarre. For example, a doctor confronted with what he believed was an inflammation of the reproductive organs might try to "draw away" the inflammation by creating what he thought were counter-irritations—blisters or sores on the groin or the thighs. The common medical practice of bleeding by means of leeches also took on some very peculiar forms in the hands of gynecologists. Dr. F. Hollick, speaking of methods of curing amenorrhea (chronic lack of menstrual periods), commented: "Some authors speak very highly of the good effects of leeches, applied to the external lips [of the genitals], a few days before the period is expected." Leeches on the breasts might prove effective too, he observed, because of the deep sympathy between the sexual organs. In some cases leeches were even applied to the cervix despite the danger of their occasional loss in the uterus. (So far as we know, no doctor ever considered perpetrating similar medical insults to the male organs.)

Such methods could be dismissed as well intentioned, if somewhat prurient, experimentation in an age of deep medical ignorance. But there were other "treatments" that were far more sinister—those aimed at altering female *behavior*. The least physically destructive of these was based, simply, on isolation and uninterrupted rest. This was used to treat a host of problems diagnosed as "nervous disorders."

Passivity was the main prescription, along with warm baths,

cool baths, abstinence from animal foods and spices, and indulgence in milk and puddings, cereals, and "mild sub-acid fruits." Women were to have a nurse—not a relative—to care for them, to receive no visitors, and as Dr. Dirix wrote, "all sources of mental excitement should be perseveringly guarded against." Charlotte Perkins Gilman was prescribed this type of treatment by Dr. S. Weir Mitchell, who advised her to put away all her pens and books. Gilman later described the experience in the story "The Yellow Wallpaper," in which the heroine, a would-be writer, is ordered by her physician-husband to "rest":

> So I take phosphates or phosphites—whichever it is, and tonics and journeys, and air, and exercise, and am absolutely forbidden to "work" until I am well again.
>
> Personally, I disagree with their ideas.
>
> Personally, I believe that congenial work, with excitement and change, would do me good.
>
> But what is one to do?
>
> I did write for a while—in spite of them; but it *does* exhaust me a good deal—having to be so sly about it. . . .or else meet with heavy opposition.

Slowly Gilman's heroine begins to lose her grip ("It is getting to be a great effort for me to think straight. Just this nervous weakness, I suppose.") and finally she frees herself from her prison—into madness, crawling in endless circles about her room, muttering about the wallpaper.

But it was the field of gynecological surgery that provided the most brutally direct medical treatments of female "personality disorders." And the surgical approach to female psychological problems had what was considered a solid theoretical basis in the theory of the "psychology of the ovary." After all, if a woman's entire personality was dominated by her reproductive organs, then gynecological surgery was the most logical approach to any female psychological problem. Beginning in the late 1860s, doctors began to act on this principle.

At least one of their treatments probably *was* effective: surgical removal of the clitoris as a cure for sexual arousal. A medical book of this period stated: "Unnatural growth of the clitoris . . . is likely to lead to immorality as well as to serious disease . . .

amputation may be necessary." Although many doctors frowned on the practice of removing the clitoris, they tended to agree that this might be necessary in cases of "nymphomania." (The last clitorectomy we know of in the United States was performed twenty-five years ago on a child of five, as a cure for masturbation.)

More widely practiced was the surgical removal of the ovaries—ovariotomy, or "female castration." Thousands of these operations were performed from 1860 to 1890. In his article "The Spermatic Economy," Ben Barker-Benfield describes the invention of the "normal ovariotomy," or removal of ovaries for non-ovarian conditions—in 1872 by Dr. Robert Battey of Rome, Georgia.

> Among the indications were a troublesomeness, eating like a ploughman, masturbation, attempted suicide, erotic tendencies, persecution mania, simple "cussedness," and dysmenorrhea. Most apparent in the enormous variety of symptoms doctors took to indicate castration was a strong current of sexual appetitiveness on the part of women.

Patients were often brought in by their husbands, who complained of their unruly behavior. When returned to their husbands, "castrated," they were "tractable, orderly, industrious and cleanly," according to Dr. Battey. (Today ovariotomy, accompanying a hysterectomy, for example, is not known to have these effects on the personality. One can only wonder what, if any, personality changes Dr. Battey's patients really went through.) Whatever the effects, some doctors claimed to have removed from fifteen hundred to two thousand ovaries; in Barker-Benfield's words, they "handed them around at medical society meetings on plates like trophies."

We could go on cataloging the ludicrous theories, the lurid cures, but the point should be clear: late nineteenth-century medical treatment of women made very little sense as *medicine*, but it was undoubtedly effective at keeping certain women—those who could afford to be patients—in their place. As we have seen, surgery was often performed with the explicit goal of "taming" a high-strung woman, and whether or not the surgery itself was

effective, the very threat of surgery was probably enough to bring many women into line. Prescribed bed rest was obviously little more than a kind of benign imprisonment—and the prescriptions prohibiting intellectual activity speak for themselves!

But these are just the extreme "cures." The great majority of upper-middle-class women were never subjected to gynecological surgery or long-term bed rest, yet they too were victims of the prevailing assumptions about women's "weakness" and the necessity of frequent medical attention. The more the doctors "treated," the more they lured women into seeing themselves as sick. The entire mystique of female sickness—the house calls, the tonics and medicines, the health spas—served, above all, to keep a great many women busy at the task of doing nothing. Even among middle-class women who could not afford constant medical attention and who did not have the leisure for full-time invalidism, the myth of female frailty took its toll, with cheap (and often dangerous) patent medicines taking the place of high-priced professional "cures."

One very important effect of all this was a great increase in the upper-middle-class woman's dependence on men. To be sure, the leisured lady of the "better" classes was already financially dependent on her husband. But the cult of invalidism made her seem dependent for her very physical survival on both her doctor and her husband. She might be tired of being a kept woman, she night yearn for a life of meaning and activity, but if she was convinced that she was seriously sick or in danger of becoming so, would she dare to break away? How could she even survive on her own, without the expensive medical care paid for by her husband? Ultimately, she might even become convinced that her restlessness was itself "sick"—just further proof of her need for a confined, inactive life. And if she did overcome the paralyzing assumption of women's innate sickness and begin to act in unconventional ways, a doctor could always be found to prescribe a return to what was considered normal.

In fact, the medical attention directed at these women amounted to what may have been a very effective surveillance system. Doctors were in a position to detect the first signs of

rebelliousness, and to interpret them as symptoms of a "disease"
which had to be "cured."

SUBVERTING THE SICK ROLE

It would be a mistake to assume that women were merely the
passive victims of a medical reign of terror. In some ways, they
were able to turn the sick role to their own advantage, especially
as a form of birth control. For the "well-bred" woman to whom
sex really *was* repugnant, and yet a "duty," or for any woman who
wanted to avoid pregnancy, "feeling sick" was a way out—and
there were few others. Contraceptive methods were virtually
unavailable; abortion was risky and illegal. It would never have
entered a respectable doctor's head to advise a lady on contraception (if he *had* any advice to offer, which is unlikely), or to offer to
perform an abortion (at least according to AMA propaganda). In
fact, doctors devoted considerable energy to "proving" that contraception and abortion were inherently unhealthy, and capable
of causing such diseases as cancer. (This was before the pill!) But
a doctor *could* help a woman by supporting her claims to be too
sick for sex: he could recommend abstinence. So who knows how
many of this period's drooping consumptives and listless invalids
were actually well women, feigning illness to escape intercourse
and pregnancy?

If some women resorted to sickness as a means of birth—and
sex—control, others undoubtedly used it to gain attention and a
limited measure of power within their families. Today, everybody
is familiar with the (sexist) myth of the mother-in-law whose
symptoms conveniently strike during family crises. In the
nineteenth century, women developed, in epidemic numbers, an
entire syndrome which even doctors sometimes interpreted as a
power grab rather than a genuine illness. The new disease was
hysteria, which in many ways epitomized the cult of female
invalidism. It affected upper- and upper-middle-class women almost exclusively; it had no discernible organic basis; and it was
totally resistant to medical treatment. For those reasons alone, it
is worth considering in some detail.

A contemporary doctor described the hysterical fit this way:

The patient . . . loses the ordinary expression of countenance, which is replaced by a vacant stare; becomes agitated; falls if before standing; throws her limbs about convulsively; twists the body into all kinds of violent contortions; beats her chest; sometimes tears her hair; and attempts to bite herself and others; and, though a delicate woman, evinces a muscular strength which often requires four or five persons to restrain her effectually.

Hysteria appeared, not only as fits and fainting, but in every other form: hysterical loss of voice, loss of appetite, hysterical coughing or sneezing, and, of course, hysterical screaming, laughing, and crying. The disease spread wildly, yet almost exclusively in a select clientele of urban middle- and upper-middle-class white women between the ages of fifteen and forty-five.

Doctors became obsessed with this "most confusing, mysterious and rebellious of diseases." In some ways, it was the ideal disease for the doctors: it was never fatal, and it required an almost endless amount of medical attention. But it was not an ideal disease from the point of view of the husband and family of the afflicted woman. Gentle invalidism had been one thing; violent fits were quite another. So hysteria put the doctors on the spot. It was essential to their professional self-esteem either to find an organic basis for the disease, and cure it, or to expose it as a clever charade.

There was plenty of evidence for the latter point of view. With mounting suspicion, the medical literature began to observe that hysterics never had fits when alone, and only when there was something soft to fall on. One doctor accused them of pinning their hair in such a way that it would fall luxuriantly when they fainted. The hysterical "type" began to be characterized as a "petty tyrant" with a "taste for power" over her husband, servants, and children, and, if possible, her doctor.

In historian Carroll Smith-Rosenberg's interpretation, the doctor's accusations had some truth to them: the hysterical fit, for many women, must have been the only acceptable outburst—of rage, of despair, or simply of *energy*—possible. But as a form of revolt it was very limited. No matter how many women might adopt it, it remained completely individualized: hysterics don't unite and fight. As a power play, throwing a fit might give a brief psychological advantage over a husband or a doctor, but ulti-

mately it played into the hands of the doctors by confirming their notion of women as irrational, unpredictable, and diseased.

On the whole, however, doctors did continue to insist that hysteria was a real disease—a disease of the uterus, in fact. (Hysteria comes from the Greek word for uterus.) They remained unshaken in their conviction that their own house calls and high physician's fees were absolutely necessary; yet at the same time, in their treatment and in their writing, doctors assumed an increasingly angry and threatening attitude. One doctor wrote, "It will sometimes be advisable to speak in a decided tone, in the presence of the patient, of the necessity of shaving the head, or of giving her a cold shower bath, should she not be soon relieved." He then gave a "scientific" rationalization for this treatment by saying, "The sedative influence of fear may allay, as I have known it to do, the excitement of the nervous centers."

Carroll Smith-Rosenberg writes that doctors recommended suffocating hysterical women until their fits stopped, beating them across the face and body with wet towels, and embarrassing them in front of family and friends. She quotes Dr. F. C. Skey: "Ridicule to a woman of sensitive mind, is a powerful weapon . . . but there is not an emotion equal to fear and the threat of personal chastisement. . . . They will listen to the voice of authority." The more women became hysterical, the more doctors became punitive toward the disease; and at the same time, they began to see the disease everywhere themselves until they were diagnosing every independent act by a woman, especially a women's rights action, as "hysterical."

With hysteria, the cult of female invalidism was carried to its logical conclusion. Society had assigned affluent women to a life of confinement and inactivity, and medicine had justified this assignment by describing women as innately sick. In the epidemic of hysteria, women were both accepting their inherent "sickness" *and* finding a way to rebel against an intolerable social role. Sickness, having become a way of life, became a way of rebellion, and medical treatment, which had always had strong overtones of coercion, revealed itself as frankly and brutally repressive.

But hysteria is more than a bizarre twist of medical history. The nineteenth-century epidemic of hysteria had lasting significance

because it ushered in a totally new "scientific" approach to the medical management of women.

While the conflict between women and their doctors in America was escalating on the issue of hysteria, Sigmund Freud, in Vienna, was beginning to work on a treatment that would remove the disease altogether from the arena of gynecology. In one stroke, he solved the problem of hysteria and marked out a new medical specialty. "Psychoanalysis," as Carroll Smith-Rosenberg has said, "is the child of the hysterical woman." Freud's cure was based on changing the rules of the game: in the first place, by eliminating the issue of whether or not the woman was faking. Psychoanalysis, as Thomas Szasz has pointed out, insists that "malingering *is* an illness—in fact, an illness 'more serious' than hysteria." Secondly, Freud established that hysteria was a mental disorder. He banished the traumatic "cures" and legitimized a doctor-patient relationship based solely on talking. His therapy urged the patient to confess her resentments and rebelliousness, and then at last to accept her role as a woman.

Under Freud's influence, the scalpel for the dissection of female nature eventually passed from the gynecologist to the psychiatrist. In some ways, psychoanalysis represented a sharp break with the past and a genuine advance for women: it was not physically injurious, and it did permit women to have sexual feelings (although only vaginal sensations were believed to be normal for adult women; clitoral sensation was "immature" and "masculine"). But in important ways, the Freudian theory of female nature was in direct continuity with the gynecological view which it replaced. It held that the female personality was inherently defective, this time due to the absence of a penis, rather than to the presence of the domineering uterus. Women were still "sick," and their sickness was still totally predestined by their anatomy.

BIBLIOGRAPHY

Barker-Benfield, Ben. "The Spermatic Economy; A Nineteenth-Century View of Sexuality," *Feminist Studies* 1, no. 1 (Summer 1972).

Cott, Nancy F., ed. *Root of Bitterness: Documents of the Social History of American Women*. New York: Dutton, 1972. See especially the section, "Sexuality and Gynecology in the Nineteenth Century."

Fruchter, Rachel Gillett. "Women's Weakness: Consumption and Women in the Nineteenth Century." Unpublished paper, 1973.

Gilman, Charlotte Perkins. *The Yellow Wallpaper*. With an afterword by Elaine R. Hedges. Old Westbury, N.Y.: The Feminist Press, 1973.

Higham, John. *Strangers in the Land: Patterns of American Nativism (1860-1925)*. New York: Atheneum, 1971. The chapter on the development of racism is full of insight into the ideological uses of "science."

Smith-Rosenberg, Carroll. "The Hysterical Woman: Sex Roles in Nineteenth-Century America," *Social Research* 39, no. 4 (Winter 1972): 652–78.

Veith, Ilza. *Hysteria: The History of a Disease*. Chicago and London: The University of Chicago Press, 1965.

Vicinus, Martha, ed. *Suffer and Be Still: Women in the Victorian Age*. Bloomington and London: Indiana University Press, 1972. A scholarly anthology ranging from menstruation to women in art.

Zaretsky, Eli. "Capitalism, the Family and Personal Life," *Socialist Revolution* 3, nos. 13 and 14 (January-April 1973): 69–125.

Nineteenth-Century Medical Books on Women

Bliss, W. W. *Woman and Her Thirty-Years' Pilgrimage*. Boston: B. B. Russell, 1870.

Clarke, Edward H., M.D. *Sex in Education, or, a Fair Chance for the Girls*. Boston: James R. Osgood and Co., 1873; reprint ed., Arno Press, 1972. The famous diatribe against higher education for women.

Dirix, M. E., M.D. *Woman's Complete Guide to Health*. New York: W. A. Townsend and Adams, 1869.

Hollick, F., M.D. *The Diseases of Woman, Their Cause and Cure Familiarly Explained*. New York: T. W. Strong, 1849.

Taylor, W. C., M.D. *A Physician's Counsels to Woman in Health and Disease*. Springfield: W. J. Holland & Co., 1871.

Warner, Lucien C., M.D. *A Popular Treatise on the Functions and Diseases of Woman*. New York: Manhattan Publishing Company, 1874.

LINDA GORDON

THE POLITICS OF BIRTH CONTROL, 1920–1940: THE IMPACT OF PROFESSIONALS

Birth control can have three major social purposes: to increase the individual freedom of women; to control overall population trends; and to improve and protect health. When the modern birth control movement began in the early twentieth century, the first was its dominant motive. Organizations demanding the legalization of birth control were formed by feminists and other radical political activists concerned with women's rights. The medical and population control motivations for supporting birth control came primarily from other sources which entered the birth control movement later but ended by dominating it.

Beginning in the 1920s birth control as a cause was taken over by male professionals, many of them physicians, in a "planned parenthood" campaign that made women's equality and autonomy a secondary issue. In the 1970s a revived feminist movement reentered the birth control cause, mainly through campaigns for legal abortion. The existence once more of an approach to birth control primarily concerned with individual human rights has created an historical context in which it is appropriate to reexamine the historical legacies behind birth control.

In this article I argue that the influx of professionals into the cause changed the goals of the birth control movement from a campaign to increase the area of self-determination for women

and all working-class people to a campaign infused with elitist values and operated in an elitist manner. These professionals were mainly of two groups: doctors and eugenists. The latter group was not, of course, a professional occupation in itself, but was mainly composed of university professors and researchers. However, professional eugenics organizations brought them together and gave them a collective consciousness as strong as that among doctors. Despite important differences, the two groups had an ultimately similar influence on birth control.

The need to identify and analyze the influence of doctors and eugenists is not merely a question of setting the historical record straight. Their impact on birth control has left serious problems today for anyone concerned with that issue. The identification of the birth control movement with the demographic theories of the population controllers and the small-family ideal of white, prosperous Americans has created antagonism to birth control among many poor people, and especially the nonwhite poor, in the United States and abroad. They often perceive population control programs as coercive, imposing alien cultural values. That antagonism to birth control is sometimes associated with an antagonism to feminism, especially since feminism until recently has been primarily a movement of educated and prosperous women. I would argue, on the contrary, that birth control has failed to cross class lines because it has not been feminist enough. A feminist birth control movement would struggle to expand women's options, to extend their right to choose, not to impose a certain economic or political theory upon them. For example, in the first agitation for birth control, feminists argued for the legitimacy of having children, in or out of marriage, and for mothers' and children's rights to a decent standard of living, as well as for women's rights not to have children.

After a brief survey of the state of the birth control movement in the early twentieth century, I will discuss first the general meaning of professionalization and then the roles of doctors and eugenists separately. There will not be space here for an evaluation of the new birth control movement that those groups created, mainly associated with Planned Parenthood, but I will offer some tentative conclusions.

THE BIRTH CONTROL MOVEMENT
IN THE EARLY TWENTIETH CENTURY

In 1915 the issue of birth control came out into the public rather suddenly, as radicals like Emma Goldman and Margaret Sanger deliberately defied obscenity laws by distributing information on contraception. By late 1916 there was a nationwide campaign of agitation and direct action for birth control. By 1917 there were national and local organizations, run almost entirely by women, devoted to the legalization of contraception. Most of these groups considered themselves within the feminist tradition, concerned with women's right to reproductive self-determination. In many instances these organizations were connected to the Socialist Party or to local socialist and anarchist groups.

Nineteenth-century feminists had argued that involuntary childbearing and child-rearing were an important cause of women's subjection. Their agitation for "voluntary motherhood,"[1] beginning in the 1870s, was limited by the prudish sexual fears and moralities that pervaded capitalist society at that time.[2] In the first decades of the twentieth century a loosening in acceptable standards of sexual conduct, particularly in the cities, made public advocacy of mechanical contraceptive devices politically possible.

Still, birth control did not immediately become respectable. Not only was it illegal, but its militant advocates were occasionally arrested on obscenity charges, though none were heavily sentenced. By the outbreak of the First World War Margaret Sanger had become the chief spokesperson for the cause. In her regular column in the *New York Call*, a Socialist Party paper, she began in 1911 to write about birth control, venereal disease, and other previously unmentionable topics. In 1914 she published seven issues of a revolutionary feminist paper, *The Woman Rebel*, which advocated birth control, printed the views of Emma Goldman, and attacked the suffrage movement for its irrelevance to working-class women. Sanger wrote that she saw birth control primarily as a means to alleviate the suffering of working-class and poor women from unwanted pregnancies, and in the long

run she identified the demand for birth control as an important weapon in the class struggle.

Rejecting the path of lobbying and winning over influential people, Sanger chose direct action. In October 1916 she, her sister, and a few other women opened a birth control clinic in Brownsville, Brooklyn. She and her sister were arrested, and the publicity around their trial and imprisonment gave them a public platform from which to present their ideas. Largely through their influence, direct action became a part of the tactics of the large network of local birth control organizations that existed by 1917.

World War I, however, brought with it a sharp and effective attack on the American Left. One of the fatalities of the rightward political swing of this period was the feminist movement. Although the woman suffrage organizations went on to victory after the war, they lost their left wing—those whose analysis of women's oppression led them to demand social change more fundamental than extension of the franchise. In 1916 the birth control activists had been politically connected to the left wing of the feminists and to profeminist groups of socialists and anarchists. When these political groupings were broken up, the birth control advocates—mostly educated women and some even upper-class—floundered politically. Losing confidence in the legitimacy of the rebellion of women of their own class, they fell back into an orientation as social workers, in the tradition of the settlement houses. Their own class position often led them to isolate the birth control issue from other social and economic pressures working-class people faced; this separation made their appeals unconvincing to the working-class women they hoped to win over. The continued existence of organized feminism might have reinforced their inclination to fight for *themselves* (as the abortion movement of the 1960s and 1970s has been powerful because it has been essentially a movement of women fighting in their own interests). Without it, the birth controllers remained social workers, with the tendency to think that they knew best what was good for their "clients." Given this orientation, it was not unnatural that the birth controllers, despite their feminism, welcomed the aid of professional experts and, in many cases, sought them out.

Of those among the original birth controllers who resisted the rightward swing of the war and postwar era, many deserted the birth control movement. For most socialists, the war itself, and then the Russian Revolution and the defense of the American Left against repression, seemed the most pressing issues after 1918. They were able to change causes because most of them had seen birth control as a reform issue rather than a revolutionary demand, something requiring less than fundamental change in the society. The tendency to distinguish between fundamental and superficial change, between revolution and reform, was characteristic of those influenced by a Marxist analysis of society. Historical and material determinism argued that certain aspects of social reality determined others, and the traditional Marxist interpretation had placed matters of sexual and reproductive relations in the "superstructure," among other cultural phenomena determined ultimately by the "substructure" which was economic relations. Liberal reformers, however, did not share this view, and several groups of professionals perceived birth control as especially fundamental. Doctors saw it as a health measure, and increasingly a preventive health measure; and naturally doctors viewed human health as a fundamental, not a superficial, condition of social progress. Eugenists saw it as a race health measure; their hereditarian views led them to consider reproduction the fundamental condition of social progress. Both groups considered reproduction fundamental, and once converted, could devote themselves to the birth control cause with passion and perseverance.

PROFESSIONALISM

Professionals entering the birth control movement brought with them a unique self-image and consciousness that made their reform work an integral part of their careers. They believed, by and large, that they worked not only to earn a living but simultaneously to help humanity, to improve society. Since they saw the content of their work as important, not merely its function in earning wages, they saw unity between their paid work and their

volunteer activities. Clearly, this view is produced by the opportunity professionals have to do creative, self-directed work. There is no mystery about the relative absence of this consciousness among working-class people or businessmen. The professional attitude toward work is largely dependent on not being paid by the hour and, for higher professionals, on the opportunity to determine their own work schedules. Furthermore, many of the professionals active in birth control, particularly doctors, were not wage workers at all, but self-employed. For both kinds of professionals—employed and self-employed—participation in reform activities if respectable enough could add to their prestige in their vocation and among their colleagues.

The desire to make a contribution to civilization led many professionals to go beyond their places of employment to seek wider social influence. For many professionals, seeking political influence seemed a contribution, not an indulgence, because they believed society needed them. Especially in the early twentieth century, many professionals believed that their superior intelligence and education entitled them to a larger share of political leadership than their numbers in the population would automatically create in a true democracy. Their review of democracy was meritocratic. Edward L. Thorndike, a eugenist educator, wrote in 1920: "The argument for democracy is not that it gives power to men without distinction, but that it gives greater freedom for ability and character to attain power!"[3] Henry Goddard, who introduced the intelligence test in the United States, thought that democracy was "a method for arriving at a truly benevolent aristocracy."[4]

Behind these politics was, first of all, the assumption that superior intelligence and education were coincident with superior political virtue. Hereditarian analyses of the causes of crime supported this view—from the theory that feeble-mindedness was a major cause of crime, to the more general attitude that if crime flowed from poverty, poverty in turn was caused by lesser ability or laziness. Professional psychologists in the 1920s were engaged in developing intelligence tests, and the bias of these tests was consistently hereditarian and meritocratic: they measured ability

to solve the kinds of problems urban professionals met with the kinds of solutions urban professionals would approve. Indeed, the Stanford-Binet test—for years the standard—classified intelligence in terms of what was "required" for five occupational groupings, the professions considered the highest. (The remaining were semiprofessional work, skilled labor, semiskilled labor, and unskilled labor, in descending order.)[5]

Professionals did not assume that their intellectual superiority came entirely from innate ability. On the contrary, they perceived that rigorous training in intellectual discipline, general knowledge, and tested methodologies had given them skills unavailable to the masses. They did not see their monopolization of this expertise and knowledge as special privilege because they were committed to equal opportunity. They did not usually perceive the effective social and economic barriers that kept most people from these opportunities. But they never doubted that their expertise and knowledge were useful guides for social policy. They did not hesitate to build professional organizations, institutions, and programs of self-licensing which excluded others from their privileges and influence, because they had confidence in the universality, objectivity, and social value of the expertise they possessed. Conscious, many of them, of having rejected aristocratic and plutocratic values, they did not think that their meritocratic values were antisocial or unjust. Their basic assumption was that greater intellectual ability, learned and innate, should be rewarded and entrusted with public power.

In the birth control movement, professionals behaved much as they did throughout the society. They sought to solve what had previously been ethical and political questions by objective study. In order to lend their support or even their names to the cause, they needed to be satisfied that it was honest, its strategies careful, and its tactics appropriate to their dignity. Even inside of voluntary associations, therefore, they distrusted leaders who did not share their own values, skills, and social status. Inevitably, their influence transformed birth control leagues from participatory membership associations into staff organizations.

Had the professionals merely changed the structure and

methods of the birth control movement, their influence could not have worked. Structure and methods in social movements cannot be separated from goals. Despite their posture as reformers who sought changes for the benefit of the whole society, or for the less fortunate in it, in fact professional men brought to the birth control movement their own political beliefs and social needs. Molded by professional training and practice but also by class origin and individual experiences, these beliefs were by no means identical among professionals and even within one profession. But leading professionals shared a common set of values, with meritocracy at its root. The professionals of the 1920s believed that some individuals were more valuable to society than others. Whether environmentalists or hereditarians or both, they doubted that superior individuals were equally distributed within all classes and ethnic groups, and believed that scientific study could determine where talent was most likely to be born. Birth control appealed to them as a means of lowering birth rates *selectively* among those groups less likely to produce babies of great merit.

Professionals also perceived themselves as social benefactors, eager not just to legalize birth control for themselves and their wives, but anxious also to install it as social policy. Their commitment to individual liberty was tempered by their recognition that some people were wiser than others, and that good social policy would not necessarily result from allowing each individual to make private decisions about such matters as birth control. Furthermore, many professionals were placed by their jobs in positions of influencing people—doctors, social workers, educators, and psychologists, for example. Accepting meritocratic political views, they naturally taught them to others. They not only disapproved of but feared a democracy that meant that all individuals, despite their educational or intellectual qualifications, would have equal power in the society; they genuinely feared the unfortunate political decisions that might result. Goddard wrote in 1920: "The disturbing fear is that the masses—the seventy or even eighty-six million—will take matters into their own hands." Rather, he argues, they should be directed by the

four million of superior intelligence.[6] This self-conscious elitism reflected not only fear but also an effort to reassure themselves of their differences from the "masses."

DOCTORS

Most physicians remained opposed to contraception in the early 1920s. The predominant position among prestigious doctors was not merely disapproval, but revulsion so hysterical that it prevented them from accepting facts. As late as 1925 Morris Fishbein, editor of the *Journal of the American Medical Association*, asserted that there were no safe and effective birth control methods.[7]

In 1926 Frederick McCann wrote that birth control had an insidious influence on the female, causing many ailments previously regarded as obscure in their origins; and that while "biology teaches" that the primary purpose of the sexual act is to reproduce, the seminal fluid also has a necessary and healthful local and general effect on the female.[8] Many doctors believed that they had a social and moral responsibility to fight the social degeneration that birth control represented. George Kosmak, a prominent gynecologist, asked rhetorically: "Is this movement to be ascribed to an honest intent to better the world, is it another expression of the spread of feministic doctrines . . . or is it merely another instance of one of those hysterical waves with which our civilization is so frequently assailed?"[9] The social values underlying Kosmak's opposition were extremely conservative:

> Fear of conception has been an important factor in the virtue of many unmarried girls, and . . . many boys are likewise kept straight by this means . . . the freedom with which this matter is now discussed . . . must have an unfortunate effect on the morals of our young people. It is particularly important . . . to keep such knowledge from our girls and boys, whose minds and bodies are not in a receptive frame for such information.

Running throughout Kosmak's attack was an expression of strong elitism:

> Those classes of our social system who are placed in a certain

position by wealth or mental attainments, require for their upkeep and regeneration the influx of individuals from the strata which are ordinarily regarded as of a lower plane . . . it is necessary for the general welfare and the maintenance of an economic balance that we have a class of the population that shall be characterized by "quantity" rather than by "quality." In other words, we need the "hewers of wood and the drawers of water" and I can only repeat the question that I have already proposed to our good friends who believe in small families, that if the "quantity" factor in our population were diminished as the result of their efforts, would they be willing to perform certain laborious tasks themselves which they now relegate to their supposed inferiors? Might I ask whether the estimable lady who considered it an honor to be arrested as a martyr to the principles advocated by Mrs. Sanger, would be willing to dispose of her own garbage at the river front rather than have one of the "quantity" delegated to this task for her?[10]

Kosmak's concern to guard accustomed privilege also applied to the particular prerogatives of his profession, and reflected the professional ideology that expertise should decide social values:

The pamphlets which have received the stamp of authority by this self-constituted band of reformers . . . are a mixture of arrant nonsense, misinformation, false reports, and in addition, in some cases, seditious libels on the medical profession. These publications are not scientific and in most instances have been compiled by non-scientific persons. . . . Efforts to impress the public with their scientific character need hardly be dignified by further professional comment, and yet they are a source of such potential danger that as physicians we must lend our assistance in doing away with what is essentially indecent and obscene. . . . Shall we permit the prescribing of contraceptive measures and drugs, many of which are potentially dangerous, by non-medical persons, when we have so jealously guarded our legal rights as physicians against Christian Scientists, osteopaths, chiropractors, naturopaths and others who have attempted to invade the field of medical practice by a short cut without sufficient preliminary training such as is considered essential for the equipment of every medical man? Will we not by mere acquiescence favor the establishment of another school of practice, the "contraceptionists," . . . if as physicians we do not raise our voices against the propaganda which is spreading like a slimy monster into our homes, our firesides, and among our young people?[11]

In protecting his profession Kosmak was very like a craft unionist. But in his sense of responsibility for morality, his point of view was uniquely professional. The sexual values that the anti-birth-control doctors cherished were not so different from nineteenth-century conservative values: that the major function of women and sexual intercourse both was reproduction of the species; that the male sex drive is naturally greater than the female, an imbalance unfortunately but probably inevitably absorbed by prostitution; that female chastity is necessary to protect the family and its descent; and that female chastity must be enforced with severe social and legal sanctions, among which fear of pregnancy functioned effectively and naturally.

Toward medical birth control.   A significant minority of physicians, however, did not share these conservative values. Arguments for a higher valuation of human sexuality as an activity in itself, separate from reproduction, were expressed not only by radicals such as Dr. William Josephus Robinson but by liberal physicians as well in the early 1920s. A leading spokesman of this point of view among prestigious physicians was gynecologist Robert Latou Dickinson. He had applied his medical expertise to social problems for several decades already. He believed that mutual sexual satisfaction was essential to happy marriage. He shared the view of Kosmak and the anti-birth-controllers that doctors ought to assert moral leadership, but chose a more flexible approach. Dickinson encouraged his Ob-Gyn colleagues to take greater initiatives as marriage and sex counsellors. In his 1920 address as President of the American Gynecological Society he recommended that the group take an interest in sociological problems. He, too, disliked the radical and unscientific associations of the birth control movement. But unlike Kosmak he preferred to respond not by ignoring the movement but by taking it over, and he urged his colleagues to that strategy as early as 1916.[12]

Sensitive to the difficulties of pulling his recalcitrant colleagues into a more liberal view of contraception, Dickinson began his campaign with a typical professional gambit. In 1923 he organized a medical group to *study* contraception, with the aim of producing the first scientific and objective evaluation of its effectiveness and safety. He consciously used antiradicalism to win

support for the plan. "May I ask you . . . whether you will lend a hand toward removing the Birth Control Clinic from the propaganda influence of the American Birth Control League . . . ," he wrote to a potential supporter in 1925.[13] So firm was Dickinson's insistence that the group would merely study, without preformed opinion, that he was able to get Kosmak himself to serve on the committee. He got financial support from wealthy Gertrude Minturn Pinchot and a qualified endorsement from the New York Obstetrical Society.

Dickinson did not merely *use* antiradicalism; it was in part his genuine purpose. His Committee on Maternal Health (CMH), as his "study" project was called, was a reaction to Margaret Sanger's efforts to open and maintain a birth control clinic.[14] Continuing her search for medical acceptance, when she planned a second clinic beginning in 1921 she projected it primarily as a center for the medical study of contraception; the women who would receive contraception would be its research subjects. When it opened in January 1923, she called it the Clinical Research Bureau. It had a physician as its supervisor, but she was a woman, not a gynecologist but formerly employed as a public health officer by the state of Georgia—in other words, she did not have professionally impressive credentials. Furthermore, Sanger had insisted on considering social and economic problems as sufficient indications for prescribing contraception. Thus because of Sanger's alternative, many doctors, while remaining suspicious of birth control, supported Dickinson's endeavor as a lesser evil.

At first Dickinson's group was hostile to the Sanger clinic. They tried to get Sanger and Dr. Bocker, head of the Clinical Research Bureau, to accept the supervision of a panel of medical men, but failed. In 1925 Dickinson wrote a report scathingly critical of the value of Bocker's scientific work.[15] But several factors intervened to lessen this hostility and even bridge the gap between Sanger and the Committee on Maternal Health. One was the fact that the CMH clinic found it difficult to get enough patients with medical indications for contraception. The CMH insistence on avoiding publicity and open endorsement of birth control made women reluctant to try the clinic, anticipating rejection and/or moralistic condemnation of their desire for birth control. Fur-

thermore, it was still extremely difficult to obtain diaphragms, which had to be smuggled into the country. By 1926, three years of work had produced only 124 incomplete case histories. Meanwhile, Sanger's clinic saw 1655 patients in 1925 alone, with an average of three visits each.[16]

Another factor leading toward unity between the two clinics was Sanger's conciliatory, even humble, attitude toward Dickinson and other influential doctors. The American Birth Control League (ABCL), which united some of the local birth control leagues into a national propaganda and lobbying staff organization, primarily under Sanger's control throughout the 1920s, had been courting medical endorsement since its establishment in 1921. The League accumulated massive medical mailing lists, for example, and sent out reprints of pro-birth-control articles from medical journals.[17] Sanger got her millionaire husband to pay a $10,000 yearly salary to a doctor, James F. Cooper, to tour the country speaking to medical groups for the ABCL.[18] Although even he was not immune from attacks as a quack,[19] he commanded the attention of male physicians as no woman agitator could ever have done. And Cooper's prestige was enhanced by sharing the speakers' platform with prestigious European physicians at the International Birth Control Conference held in New York in 1925 under ABCL auspices. Indeed, the prestige of the Europeans—whose medical establishment was far more enlightened on the birth control question than was the American—was sufficient to entice the president of the American Medical Association, William A. Pusey, to offer a lukewarm endorsement of birth control at that conference.[20] The ABCL kept exhaustive files, not only of letters but also from their clipping service, on every physician who appeared even mildly favorable to birth control. By 1927 they had 5484 names.[21] Sanger's standard procedure in response to letters asking for information on contraceptives was to send the writer the names of nearby sympathetic doctors. In response to criticism of her clinic from the Dickinson group in 1925, Sanger, avoiding any defensive reaction, asked the Committee on Maternal Health to take over and run the clinic, hoping in return to be able to get licensing from the New York State Board of Charities. Dickinson de-

manded in return the removal of all propagandistic literature and posters, to which Sanger agreed. The scheme failed anyway, because Sanger's radical reputation, and opposition from the Catholic Church, led the State Board to refuse a license.[22] Dickinson, on the other hand, made his professional influence clear and useful to Sanger by procuring for her a $10,000 grant from the Rockefeller-backed Bureau of Social Hygiene.

Undoubtedly the largest single factor drawing doctors into the birth control movement, however, was Sanger's support for a "doctors only" type of birth control legislation, legislation that would simply strike out all restrictions on doctors' rights to prescribe contraception, giving them unlimited discretion. A corollary to Sanger's support for federal and state "doctors only" bills was her work on birth control conferences at which nonmedical personnel were excluded from the sessions which discussed the technique of contraception. At birth control conferences in 1921 and 1925 organized by the ABCL, sessions on contraception were for physicians only and by invitation only.

Meanwhile, other birth control groups, such as the Voluntary Parenthood League, continued to campaign for open bills, exempting discussion of contraception from all restrictions for anyone. These groups had substantial objections to the "doctors only" bill. In a letter to members of the Voluntary Parenthood League, President Myra Gallert wrote:

> Yes, of course we believe in medical advice for the individual, but again how about the large mass of women who cannot reach even a clinic? . . . Mrs. Sanger's own pamphlet on methods finds its way through the American mails . . . *and it is not a physician's compilation* . . . Mrs. Sanger herself testified "that the Clinical Research Department of the American Birth Control League teaches methods so simple that once learned, any mother who is intelligent enough to keep a nursing bottle clean, can use them."[23]

Furthermore, the "doctors only" bills left "the whole subject" . . . still in the category of crime and indecency.[24] Not only did they accept the definition of sexuality without reproduction as obscene, but they also removed the technique of birth control from a woman's own control. If women could not have

direct access to birth control information, they would have to get their information from doctors, accompanied by censorship at worst and moral guidance at best.

Tactically, the "doctors only" bill also had serious repercussions. As Dr. Antoinette Konikow wrote, the very advantage that its supporters liked—that it would make birth control seem safely controlled—was its worst feature "because it emasculates enthusiasm. To the uninformed the exemption seems hardly worth fighting for."[25] The very substance of the politics doctors brought to the birth control movement tended to squash widespread participation in the movement.

Many doctors, of course, believed that they had weighty reasons to oppose an "open bill." Sharing the views expressed by Kosmak in 1917, their sense of professional responsibility and importance led them to anticipate all sorts of moral and physiologic disasters should contraceptive information and devices be generally available.

A local birth control league: the Massachusetts case. The effect of concentration on a "doctors only" bill can be seen by examining the work of a local birth control league. While there were of course many differences in the histories of the local leagues, we are emphasizing here certain developments that were common to most of them while illustrating them with specifics from the Massachusetts case. A birth control group had emerged in Boston in 1916 with the arrest of a young male agitator, a Fabian socialist, for giving a police agent a pamphlet entitled "Why and How the Poor Should Not Have Many Children." Supporters of the accused, Van Kleeck Allison, organized a defense committee which later became the Birth Control League of Massachusetts (BCLM). The League members were from the beginning a coalition of radicals (Allison's fellow Fabians and members of local Socialist Party groups) and liberals (social workers and eugenics reformers in particular). As elsewhere, no doctors—with the exception of the revolutionary socialist Dr. Antoinette Konikow—were conspicuous in the movement in its first years.[26]

The BCLM members agreed in 1916 and 1917 on tactics designed to make birth control a public issue and a popular cause.

They tried and often succeeded in getting publicity in the popular press, they held mass meetings and public debates, and they contacted 900 women's clubs around the state in efforts to recruit supporters. They accepted support from all quarters, and featured speakers identified as radicals. From the beginning, however, some of the socialists in the BCLM encountered a tension between offering a genuinely radical social alternative and using the support of conservative but powerful people to win immediate gains. Cerise Carman Jack, a Harvard faculty wife of radical leanings, expressed her conflicts about the tension between her radical ideas and her desire to win:

It is the same old and fundamental question that everyone who has any independence of mind encounters as soon as he tries to support a really radical movement by the contributions of the conservative. . . . The Settlements have . . . found it out and have become . . . crystallized around activities of a noncreative sort; the politician has found it out and is for the most part content to lose his soul in the game. . . . [But] half-baked radicals . . . [tend to] have nothing to do with any movement that savors of popularity and . . . think that all reforms must be approached by the narrow path of martyrdom.[27]

Cerise Jack was typical of many women of similar views when she decided in 1918 that the most important and strategic direction for her political efforts should be defense work against political repression. Birth control could wait; it would come anyway after the revolution, would "come so spontaneously wherever the radicals get control of the government, just as the war has brought suffrage . . . now is the time to work for the fundamentals and not for reform measures."[28]

In Massachusetts, as in many places, the immediate effect of the defection of radicals and the entrance of professionals into the Birth Control League was a period of inactivity. In 1918, birth control supporters among high professionals were still the minority. Most doctors, lawyers, ministers, and professors found birth control too radical and improper a subject for public discussion. Besides, they feared "race suicide" among their own class. But throughout the 1920s quiet but steady concentration on a "doctors only" bill by remaining birth control activists transformed

medical opinion. Despite Massachusetts' special problem of strong Catholic pressure against birth control, the League got 1200 doctors to endorse its bill.[29] The principle of doctors' rights even led the by now exclusively liberal and conservative Massachusetts Birth Control League to defend radical Dr. Antoinette Konikow. She regularly lectured on sex hygiene to women, demonstrating contraceptives as she discussed birth control, and was arrested for this on February 9, 1928. She appealed to the now defunct League and her defense in fact rehabilitated the League under its old president, Blanche Ames Ames. Konikow was a difficult test case for the League to accept: a Bolshevik and a regular contributor to revolutionary socialist periodicals, she lacked a refined personal style and was rumored to be an abortionist. Nevertheless, the principle at stake was too important for the doctors to ignore: the prosecution of any physician under the obscenity statutes would have set a dangerous precedent for all physicians. The Emergency Defense Committee formed for Konikow worked out an extremely narrow line of defense: that she was not exhibiting contraceptive devices within the meaning of the law but was using them to illustrate a scientific lecture and warn against possible injuries to health.[30] This line worked and Konikow was acquitted.

The verdict stimulated renewed birth control activity and a new BCLM nucleus drew together with the goal of persuading doctors to support birth control and passing a "doctors only" bill in Massachusetts. A new board for the BCLM was chosen, and ten of the sixteen new members were physicians. The lobbying activities took all the League's time, and there was virtually no public visibility in this period. Konikow herself was extremely critical of this policy. She saw that commitment to it required maintaining a low profile and specifically meant giving up the project of a clinic. She argued, in fact, that opening a clinic would in the long run do more to bring the medical profession around than a long, slow legislative lobbying campaign.[31] Konikow's criticisms angered the League people. Possibly in retaliation, they refused to lend her the League mailing list of 1500 names to publicize her new book, *The Physicians' Manual of Birth Control*. Konikow's angry protests condemned what she

saw as a new kind of organization quite different from that of the original local birth control leagues: "the relations between the Executive Board and the membership are so distant that the members do not know what the official policy of the organization is . . ."[32]

As Konikow had predicted, one of the consequences of this new kind of organization was failure. While the BCLM had become narrow and elitist, the opposition from the Catholic Church was based on mass support. The Birth Control League, meanwhile, had become less an organization than a professionals' lobbying group. Furthermore, no matter how decorous and conservative the League's arguments for birth control, they could not escape red-baiting and other forms of scurrilous attack. Cardinal O'Connell said that the bill was a "direct threat . . . towards increasing impurity and unchastity not only in our married life but . . . among our unmarried people . . ." The chief of obstetrics at a Catholic hospital said that the bill was "the essence and odor that comes from that putrid and diseased river that has its headquarters in Russia." Another opponent made the direct charge that this was a campaign supported by Moscow gold.[33] A broad opposition defeated the doctors' bill. Even non-Catholic attackers recognized the radical potential of birth control: separation of sex from reproduction, and removal of one of the main sanctions for marital chastity—involuntary pregnancy. Even had birth control never had its reputation "damaged" by association with socialists, anarchists, and Free Lovers, its content could not be disguised. This was the weak point in the conservative strategy of the BCLM, even measured against its own goals. If birth control was inherently radical, subversive of conventional morality in its *substance*, no form of persuasion could bring around those who needed and benefited from the conventional morality. The meaning of birth control could not be disguised by coating it as a medical tool.

While the Catholic Church played a particularly large role in Massachusetts, "doctors only" bills were defeated in every state in which they were proposed, even in states without large Catholic populations.[34] Indeed, the whole pattern of development of the BCLM was echoed in many local birth control leagues. After the

radical originators of the movements left because of the War and other causes that seemed to them more pressing (or, in a few instances, were pushed out by professionals and conservatives), the birth control leagues fell into much lower levels of activity and energy. The impact of professionals—particularly doctors— on birth control as a social movement was to depress it, to take it out of the mass consciousness as a social issue, even as information on contraceptives continued to be disseminated. Furthermore, the doctors did not prove successful in the 1920s even in winning the legislative and legal gains they had defined as their goals. While some birth control organizers, such as Cerise Jack of the BCLM, felt that they were torn between radical demands and effectiveness, in fact there is reason to question whether the surrender of radical demands produced any greater effectiveness at all.

The problem of clinics. The Massachusetts example, while typical of the national struggle for legislation legalizing birth control, was not representative of the development of birth control clinics. By 1930 there were fifty-five clinics in twenty-three cities in twelve states. In Chicago in 1923 a birth control clinic was denied a license by the City Health Commissioner, but the League secured a court order overruling him and granting a license. Judge Fisher's decision in this case marked out important legal precedents. His opinion held that the project was a clinic under the meaning of the law; that there existed contraceptive methods not injurious to health; that the actions of the Health Commissioner (who had cited Biblical passages in his letter of refusal to license!) amounted to enforcing religious doctrines, an illegal use of power; that the obscenity statutes only sought to repress "promiscuous" distribution of contraceptive information; and that "where reasonable minds differ courts should hesitate to condemn."[35]

As the clinic movement mushroomed around the country, however, conflict raged about how and by whom the clinics should be controlled. Margaret Sanger still resisted relinquishing personal control of her New York clinic to the medical profession. No doubt part of her resistance came from a desire to control things herself, especially since she had lost control of the

American Birth Control League and its publication, the *Birth Control Review*, by 1929. (Sanger was undoubtedly a difficult person who did not thrive on cooperative work. Her personal struggles within the birth control movement are well described in Kennedy.)[36] But part of her resistance, too, came from disagreement with the doctors' insistence on requiring medical indications for the prescription of contraceptive devices. Her Clinical Research Bureau had consistently stretched the definition of appropriate indications; and if an appropriate medical problem that justified contraception could not be found, a patient was often referred to private doctors whose prescriptions would be less dangerous.[37] Sanger was willing to avoid an open challenge to the law on the question of indications, but she was not willing to allow close medical supervision to deprive physically healthy women of access to contraception.

She still wanted a license to guarantee the safety and stability of her clinic. When she withdrew the clinic from the auspices of the ABCL in 1928, Sanger once again approached Dickinson, requesting that he find her a medical director whose prestige might help obtain a license. Dickinson in reply demanded that the clinic be entirely turned over to a medical authority, suggesting New York Hospital. Sanger was convinced that such an affiliation would hamstring her work and refused it. Then, in April 1929, the clinic was raided by the police. A plainclothes policewoman asked for and was supplied with a contraceptive device. She even came for her second checkup to make sure her diaphragm was fitting her well, and then returned five days later with a detachment of police who arrested three nurses and two physicians, and confiscated the medical records. The last action was a mistake on the part of the police, for it could not help but unite the medical profession behind Sanger, in defense of confidential medical records. Furthermore, the policewoman had been a poor choice because the clinic doctors had indeed found pelvic abnormalities that provided a proper medical indication for giving her a diaphragm. The case was thrown out of court. (Some time later the policewoman returned to the clinic, off duty, to seek treatment for her pelvic disorders!)[38]

This episode produced good feelings between Sanger and the

doctors who supported her, and Dickinson followed it up with a last attempt to persuade her to give up the clinic—this time into the hands of the New York Academy of Medicine rather than a hospital. Sanger was probably closer to acceding now than she had ever been and might have done so had it not been for countervailing pressure she was getting from another group of professionals—the eugenists. Though easily as conservative as the doctors in terms of the feminist or sexual freedom implications of birth control, they were solidly in Sanger's camp on the issue of indications. They could not be content with a medical interpretation of contraception, i.e., that its function was to prevent pathologies in mothers. The eugenists sought the kind of impact birth control might have when disseminated on a mass basis; they wanted to improve the quality of the whole population, not just protect the health of women. They also felt a certain amount of professional rivalry with the physicians. Eugenists had been among the earliest of the nonradicals to support birth control, and some of them had spoken out for it publicly even before the War. They perceived the doctors as joining the cause after it was safe, and trying to take it over from its originators.[39] Though politically conservative, their intensity of commitment to their reform panacea—selective breeding—allowed them to accept Sanger's militant rhetoric and her willingness to challenge and stretch the law. At the same time the eugenists had a great influence not only on Sanger but on the whole birth control movement.

EUGENISTS

Eugenics attitudes had attracted reformers of all varieties for nearly a century. Lacking a correct genetics, nineteenth-century eugenics was largely utopian speculations based on the assumption that acquired characteristics could be inherited. This assumption meant that there was no necessary opposition between environmentalism and heredity. The scientific discrediting of the theory of the inheritance of acquired characteristics changed the political implications of eugenics, and more narrow applications of it became dominant. Margaret Sanger described the develop-

ment of eugenics succinctly: "Eugenics, which had started long before my time, had once been defined as including free love and prevention of conception. . . . Recently it had cropped up again in the form of selective breeding."[40] The new eugenics, "selective breeding," was rigidly elitist, intended to reproduce the entire American population in the image of those who dominated it politically and economically. The "new" eugenics was not a reform program but a justification for the status quo. Its essential argument—that the "unfit," the criminal, and the pauper were the products of congenital formations—suited the desire of its upper-class supporters to justify their own monopoly on power, privilege, and wealth.

Eugenics ideology. New genetic theories provided reliable methods of prediction, and therefore control, of the transmittal of some identifiable physical traits, and they stimulated a great deal of scientific research into human genetics. The first eugenics organizations were research centers, such as the Eugenics Record Office and the Station for Experimental Evolution. As eugenics enthusiasts developed specific political and social proposals for action, they established organizations to spread the gospel generally and do legislative lobbying specifically. The first of these was the Eugenics Section of the American Breeders Association, set up in 1910, in 1913 human breeding became the main focus of the Association which changed its name to the American Genetic Association. Several other organizations were established in the next decade.

In no academic field was the coalition between corporate capital and scholars developed more fully than in eugenics. By the 1920s eugenics was a required course in many American universities. The development of eugenics as a scholarly field represented the capitulation of university scholars to a fad, allowing their skills to become a commodity for sale to a high bidder. The backers of eugenics research and writing included the wealthiest families of the country. The Eugenics Record Office was established by Mrs. E. H. Harriman.[41] The Station for Experimental Evolution was funded by Andrew Carnegie.[42] Henry Fairfield Osborn, a gentleman scholar and founder of the New York Museum of Natural History, was a main financial backer of the eugenics societies; in

the late 1920s Frederick Osborn, nephew of Henry Fairfield, assumed leadership in the cause and financed a research program for the Eugenics Research Association.[43]

Despite the direct influence of big business on eugenics, the cause carried with it some of its historic aura of radicalism for many years, an aura which sometimes disguised its fundamentally conservative content. For example, eugenists identified themselves as crusaders for reform, and argued their case with apocalyptic warnings (e.g., "race suicide," "menace to civilization") and utopian promises ("a world of supermen"). They advocated techniques, such as sterilization and marriage licensing, which were often repulsive to traditional and religious people. Equally important, many radicals remained interested in eugenics programs. Socialists, feminists, and sex-radicals continued to use eugenics ideas. Mainly outside academic and scientific circles, these followers of a traditional "popular eugenics" continued to offer analyses and proposals that assumed the inheritance of acquired characteristics well into the 1920s. They endorsed programs to lessen suffering through the prevention of birth defects; they included demands for prenatal medical care for women under the aegis of eugenics.

After the First World War, however, academic eugenists consistently avoided all except strictly hereditarian interpretations of eugenics. In clinging to their hereditarian assumptions,[44] they stood in opposition to the tradition of social reform in America. Eugenists justified social and economic inequalities as biological; their journals featured articles about "aristogenic" families, as if the existence of several noted gentlemen in the same family proved the superiority of their genes. Their definitions of what was socially worthy naturally used their own professional and upper-class standards of success. The professional bias can be seen particularly clearly in their emphasis on intelligence. Standard eugenics concepts of inferiority, such as "degeneracy," consistently equated lack of intelligence with viciousness and intelligence with goodness.[45] "Among the 1000 leading American men of science," eugenist Paul Popenoe wrote, "there is not one son of a day laborer. It takes 48,000 unskilled laborers to produce one man distinguished enough to get in *Who's Who*, while the

same number of Congregational ministers produces 6000 persons eminent enough to be included."[46]

Aristogenic stock was missing not only from the working class as a whole, but also from non-Yankees in particular. Here is a typical explanation of the problem from a standard eugenics textbook first published in 1916:

> From the rate at which immigrants are increasing it is obvious that our very life-blood is at stake. For our own protection we must face the question of what types or races should be ruled out . . . many students of heredity feel that there is great hazard in the mongreliz-ing of distinctly unrelated races. . . . However, it is certain that under existing social conditions in our own country only the most worth-less and vicious of the white race will tend in any considerable numbers to mate with the negro and the result cannot but mean deterioration on the whole for either race.[47]

Consider the following—typical—passage from *Revolt Against Civilization: The Menace of the Under Man* by Lothrop Stod-dard, one of the most widely respected eugenists:

> But what about the inferior? Hitherto we have not analyzed their attitude. We have seen that they are incapable of either creating or furthering civilization, and are thus a negative hindrance to prog-ress. But the inferiors are not mere negative factors in civilized life; they are also positive—in an inverse destructive sense. The inferior elements are, instinctively or consciously, the enemies of civiliza-tion. And they are its enemies, not by chance but because they are more or less uncivilizable.[48]

The eugenics movement strongly supported immigration re-striction,[49] and contributed to the development of racist fears and hatreds among many Americans. In 1928, the Committee on Selective Immigration of the American Eugenics Society rec-ommended that future immigration be restricted to white people.[50] The movement also supported the enactment of anti-miscegenation laws throughout the South,[51] and Southern ra-cists used the respectability of eugenics to further the develop-ment of segregation. For example, the Virginia State Board of Health distributed a pamphlet among schoolchildren entitled "Eugenics in Relation to the New Family and the Law on Racial

Integrity," published in 1924. It explained in eugenic terms the valiant and lonely effort of Virginia to preserve the race from the subversion fostered by the nineteen states plus the District of Columbia which permitted miscegenation. It concluded, "Let us turn a deaf ear to those who would interpret Christian brotherhood to mean racial equality."

Toward eugenical birth control. When they turned their attention to "positive eugenics," most eugenists were antagonistic toward birth control. To appreciate this conflict fully, one must remember that the eugenists were concerned not only with the inadequate reproduction of the "superior," but also with a declining birth rate in general. As late as 1940, demographers worried that the net reproduction rate of the United States was below the replacement level.[52] Many eugenists clung to the mercantilist notion that a healthy economy should have a steadily growing population. In addition, they adopted the "race suicide" analyses that birth control was being practiced in a particularly dysgenic way, the best "stock" producing the fewest children. In the area of "negative" eugenics, they approved of birth limitation, of course, but preferred to see it enforced more permanently—through sterilization and the prohibition of dysgenic marriages.

The feminist content of birth control practice and propaganda was especially obnoxious to the eugenists. They feared the growing "independence" of women. Eugenists were frequently involved in propaganda for the protection of the family, and in antidivorce campaigning. The most common eugenics position was virulently antifeminist, viewing women primarily as breeders. One typical eugenist wrote in 1917: "In my view, women exist primarily for racial ends. The tendency to exempt the more refined of them from the pains and anxieties of childbearing and motherhood, although arising out of a very attractive feeling of consideration for the weaker individuals of the race, is not, admirable as it seems, in essence a moral one."[53]

While most eugenists were opposed to birth control, some were not, and all saw that they had certain common interests with the birth controllers. Some believed that while sterilization would be necessary in extreme cases, birth control could be taught to and practiced by the masses. Especially the younger eugenists and the

demographer-sociologists (demography was not at this time a distinct discipline) were convinced that the trend toward smaller families was irrevocable, and that the only thing to do to counteract its dysgenic tendency was to make it universal. Finally, they shared with birth controllers an interest in sex education and freedom of speech on sexual issues.

If these factors contributed to close the gap between eugenists and birth controllers, the attitudes of the birth controllers contributed even more. While eugenists by and large opposed birth control, birth controllers did not make the reverse judgment. On the contrary, almost all birth control supporters, both leaders and followers, agreed with eugenics goals and felt that they could gain from the popularity of eugenics.

Identification with eugenics goals was, for many birth controllers, based on familiarity with the nineteenth-century radical eugenics tradition. Most of them did not immediately apprehend the transformation of eugenics by the adoption of exclusively hereditarian assumptions. Some radicals were critical of the class basis of eugenics programs, as was socialist Henry Bergen in 1920:

> Unfortunately eugenists are impelled by their education and their associations and by the unconscious but not less potent influences of the material and social interests of their class to look upon our present environment . . . as a constant factor, which not only cannot be changed but ought not to be changed. [54]

But most socialists accepted the fundamental eugenics belief in the importance of congenital characteristics. Thus British birth controller and socialist Eden Paul wrote in 1917 that the "socialist tendency is to overrate the importance of environment, great as this undoubtedly is . . ."[55] Furthermore, on issues of race or ethnic differences the Left shared with the Right deep prejudices. In the same article in which Bergen identified the class function of eugenics, he endorsed the goal of using eugenics programs to improve the white race.[56] In a socialist collection of essays on birth control published in 1917 we find passages such as this:

> Taking the coloured population in 1910 as ten millions; it would in 1930 be twenty millions; in 1950, forty millions; in 1970, eighty millions; and 1990, one hundred and sixty millions. A general pro-

hibition of white immigration would thus, within the space of about eighty years, suffice to transform the Union into a negro realm. Now, although individual members of the Afro-American race have been able, when educated by whites, to attain the highest levels of European civilisation, negroes as a whole have not hitherto proved competent to maintain a lofty civilisation. The condition of affairs in the black republic of Haiti gives some justification for the fear that negro dominance would be disastrous.[57]

Like the rest of the Left, the feminist birth controllers tended to accept racist and ethnocentric attitudes. As did most middle-class reformers, the feminists also had a reservoir of anti-working-class attitudes. The American feminist movement had its own traditions of elitism, in the style of Elizabeth Cady Stanton's proposal for suffrage for the educated.[58] Many feminists had been active in the temperance movement, and saw immigrants and working-class men as drunken undesirables. Anti-Catholicism particularly had been an undercurrent in the women's rights movement for decades, stimulated by Catholic opposition to prohibition and women's rights. Southern feminists used the fear of the black vote as an argument for suffrage, and were supported by the national women's suffrage organizations in doing so.[59] Birth control reformers were not attracted to eugenics *because* they were racists; rather, they had interests in common with eugenists and had no strong tradition of antiracism on which to base a critique of eugenics.

Sanger, too, had always argued the "racial" values of birth control, but as time progressed she gave less attention to feminist arguments and more to eugenical ones. "More children from the fit, less from the unfit—that is the chief issue of birth control," she wrote in 1919.[60] In *Woman and the New Race*,[61] published in 1920, she put together statistics about immigrants, their high birth rates, and low literacy rates in a manner certain to stimulate racist fears. In *The Pivot of Civilization*,[62] published in 1922, she urged applying stockbreeding techniques to society in order to avoid giving aid to "good-for-nothings" at the expense of the "good." She warned that the masses of the illiterate and "degenerate" might well destroy "our way of life." She developed favorite eugenical subthemes as well, such as the cost to the society of

supporting the "unfit" in public institutions, and the waste of funds on charities that merely were putting band-aids on sores rather than curing diseases. Society is divided into three demographic groups, she argued: the wealthy who already practiced birth control; the intelligent and responsible who wanted birth control; and the reckless and irresponsible, including "the pauper element dependent entirely upon the normal and fit members of society."[63] She shifted her imagery about such social divisions, for later in the 1920s she cited a "Princeton University authority" who had classified the United States population as twenty million intellectual, twenty-five million mediocre, forty-five million subnormal, and fifteen million feeble-minded.[64] The racism and virulence of her eugenical rhetoric grew most extreme in the early 1930s. In 1932 she recommended the sterilization or segregation by sex of "the whole dysgenic population."[65] She complained that the government, which was so correctly concerned with the quality of immigrants, lacked concern for the quality of its native-born.[66]

Eugenics soon became a constant, even a dominant, theme at birth control conferences. In 1921 at the organizational conference of the American Birth Control League there were many eugenics speakers and exhibits of charts showing the dysgenic heritage of the infamous Jukes and Kallikak families. In 1922 Sanger went to London for the Fifth International Neo-Malthusian and Birth Control Conference as its only female honored guest. Yet not a single panel was devoted to birth control as a woman's right nor did Sanger raise this point of view.[67] In 1925 Sanger brought the Sixth International Conference to New York under the sponsorship of the ABCL. The impact of ABCL control was to make the emphasis more eugenical and less neo-Malthusian, but there was no increase in concern with women's rights. Not a single session was chaired by a woman; about one out of ten speakers was a woman. Four of the total of eleven sessions focused specifically on eugenics, none on women's problems.[68]

Meanwhile the propaganda of the ABCL was becoming more focused on eugenics at the expense of women's rights. The introductory brochure used during the 1920s lists the first point of

"What This Organization Does to Inform the Public" as publishing and distributing literature and conducting lectures "on the disgenic [sic] effects of careless breeding." The program of the ABCL included a sterilization demand and called for "racial progress."

The *Birth Control Review*, the ABCL publication, reflected eugenics influence from its inception in 1917. While eugenists of the older radical tradition dominated in its first years, it also printed without editorial comment a eugenical anti-birth-control argument, virtually a "race suicide" argument, in its very first volume.[69] By 1920 the *Review* published openly racist articles.[70] In 1923 the *Review* editorialized in favor of immigration restriction on a racial basis.[71] In the same year the *Review* published a study on "The Cost to the State of the Socially Unfit."[72] In 1920 Havelock Ellis favorably reviewed Lothrop Stoddard's *The Rising Tide of Color Against White World-Supremacy*.[73] Stoddard was at this time on the Board of Directors of the American Birth Control League. So was C. C. Little, another openly racist eugenist. President of the Third Race Betterment Conference, he justified birth control as an antidote to the "melting pot," a means of preserving the purity of "Yankee stock."[74] Also closely involved with the ABCL and writing regularly for *Review* was Guy Irving Burch, a director of the American Eugenics Society and leader in the American Coalition of Patriotic Societies. He supported birth control, he wrote, because he had long worked to "prevent the American people from being replaced by alien or Negro stock, whether it be by immigration or by overly high birth rates among others in this country."[75] A content analysis of the *Review* showed that by the late 1920s only 4.9 percent of all its articles for a decade had had any concern with women's self-determination.[76]

The decline of a people's birth control movement. It is important to understand correctly the birth controllers' conversion to eugenics and their desertion of feminism. They did not disavow their earlier feminism so much as find it not useful because of the more general change in the country's political climate. Had they had deeper feminist or antiracist convictions, they might have found eugenics ideas more uncomfortable. But feeling no discomfort, they found eugenics ideas useful. They could get from

the eugenists a support that they never got from the Left. The men who dominated the socialist movement did not perceive birth control as fundamental to their own interests, and their theory categorized it as a reform peripheral to the struggle of the working class. Eugenists, on the other hand, once they caught on to the idea of urging birth control upon the poor rather than condemning it among the rich, were prepared to offer active and powerful support.

Nevertheless, the professionalization of the birth control movement was identical with its takeover by men. Although women remained the majority of the membership of the large birth control organizations, the officers and the clinic directors more and more frequently became men. By 1940 Margaret Sanger had been kicked upstairs to being "honorary chairman." Men came to occupy the positions of president, general director, and all the five vice-presidents. Two of them were noted eugenists and authors of explicitly racist tracts—anti-immigrant and anti-black.[77] The only remaining woman on the board was Mrs. Mary Woodard Reinhardt, secretary.

The men, however, did not all agree. While doctors and eugenists could mesh their concerns for individual and racial health in propaganda, they did not see eye to eye on the practice of the clinics. Particularly as regards indications, as we have seen, the doctors wanted to preserve narrow medical justifications for prescribing contraceptives, while eugenists and many lay birth controllers wanted to use contraception to ameliorate social, psychologic, and economic problems as well. Beyond this, eugenists were eager to use birth control clinics to collect data on family patterns, birth control use, changing attitudes, sexual behavior, and genetic history.[78] The eugenists were there in the forefront of the social sciences. Many eugenists (e.g., Lewis Terman and Edward Thorndike) were leaders in the development of improved quantitative and statistical techniques in the social sciences. The foundations generously funded such statistical studies.[79] Eugenists feared and opposed medical supervision of clinics because it threatened to interfere with their data collection.[80]

Most birth control clinics appreciated the eugenists' support

for disseminating contraceptives in the absence of pathologic indications. The clinics also acceded to eugenists' research interests. Many clinics conducted inquiries into the hereditary histories of their patients, and presumably advised the women as to the desirability of having children.[81] In 1925, responding to suggestions from her eugenist supporters, Sanger reformed her clinical records to show the nationality, heredity, religion, occupation, and even trade union affiliation of patients.[82] A review of the work of seventy birth control clinics in Britain and the United States, published in 1930, proudly demonstrated that they reached a disproportionately large number of working-class women, and claimed a eugenic effect from doing so.[83]

The birth controllers also influenced the eugenists, of course. As Sanger described the relationship:

> Eugenics without birth control seemed to me a house built upon sands. It could not stand against the furious winds of economic pressure which had buffeted into partial or total helplessness a tremendous proportion of the human race. The eugenists wanted to shift the birth control emphasis from less children for the poor to more children for the rich. We went back on that and sought first to stop the multiplication of the unfit.[84]

Thus in one paragraph is condensed the transformation of birth control politics: the poor, "buffeted into partial or total helplessness" by economic pressure, are rechristened the unfit.

With such an attitude toward the poor, it is not surprising that the clinics encountered difficulties in teaching working-class women to use birth control properly. Some such women were unteachable, Sanger and several other birth control leaders agreed. They particularly had trouble with "the affectionate, unreflecting type known to housing experts, who, though living in one room with several children, will keep a St. Bernard dog." For these women, sterilization was recommended.[85] Another area in which the snobbery of the birth control workers was manifest was in their attitude toward working-class men. They projected an image of these husbands as uncontrolled, uncontrollable, sex-hungry, violent sexual aggressors, with no regard or respect for their wives, who would never agree to contraception. Certainly

the reasons such men might have for hostility to birth control clinics were not taken seriously.

But medical supervision of the clinics had created similar problems in reaching the poor with birth control, and Sanger and other clinic partisans ultimately saw more usefulness in the propaganda of eugenics than in the more reserved, "soft sell" style of doctors. Furthermore, the eugenists could not exercise the kind of direct control over clinics that the doctors could, lacking the institutions such as hospitals or medical academies, and were thus willing to share control with birth controllers like Sanger. If Sanger and her colleagues ultimately chose to work with the eugenists, it was because it seemed to them the only realistic option. They would greatly have preferred cooperative working relationships with both groups; and perhaps, had this been possible, they might have retained more direct power in their own hands by playing off the two groups of professionals against each other. As it was, the ideological disagreements and, even more, the jurisdictional rivalry of the two professions prevented this.

Ultimately, the rivalry held back the clinic movement. Although contraception became widespread in the 1930s, most middle-class people continued to get their help from private doctors. Working-class people, on the other hand, often did not get it at all. Many studies have shown that poor people have more excess fertility—in terms of their *own* preferences—than more prosperous people.[86] It is equally clear that poor people have little access to birth control services. This last is, of course, part of the general inadequacy and unequal distribution of medical care in the United States. Poverty generally tends to limit the use of medical facilities to the treatment of emergencies and acute or painful conditions, and minimizes access to preventive health services. While the right to birth control is not a medical issue, the actual delivery of most contraceptives must be done in medical situations. The movement for birth control clinics was thus in itself a break with the private capitalist medical system in the United States, and its failure was a part of a general failure of American medicine.

Physicians' attitudes toward the birth control movement—their demand for exclusive control and restrictive distribution—

represented a microcosm of the general attitude taken by the medical profession. The attitude of many doctors toward their private patients continued, well into the mid-twentieth century, to parallel that of many elite nineteenth-century doctors: while they opposed the "promiscuous," "indiscriminate" dissemination of contraception, they did not question their own discrimination and even thought it important that private doctors should be able to make exceptions to the policies they supported as general rules. Well-to-do women were able to secure diaphragms without medical indications from doctors who may themselves have opposed making it possible for clinics to use the same principles. The discretionary right of the individual doctor was a privilege as cherished by the profession as that of privacy—and the latter, of course, protected the former.

In the 1930s eugenics went into eclipse as a mass cause. Nazi eugenic policies tarnished the image of the movement, and scientific criticisms of Galtonian genetics stripped away much of the academic respectability that had clothed eugenical racism. On the other hand, the success of birth control also contributed to the decline of eugenics.

Birth control had become a movement that could do much of the eugenists' work for them. Henry Pratt Fairchild, former President of the American Eugenics Society, told the annual meeting of the Birth Control Federation (successor to the ABCL) in 1940:

> One of the outstanding features of the present conference is the practically universal acceptance of the fact that these two great movements [eugenics and birth control] have now come to such a thorough understanding and have drawn so close together as to be almost indistinguishable. [87]

CONCLUSION

Birth control emerged as a movement in the second decade of the century among radicals, especially feminists, who sought basic social change in sexual and class relations. By the end of the 1930s birth control was no longer a popular movement but had become a staff organization of experts lobbying for reforms on behalf of a larger constituency. I have argued that this transfor-

mation was accomplished by the large-scale entrance of professionals into the birth control cause; in this article I have singled out doctors and academic eugenists, but in the book from which this is an excerpt I have also discussed the important role of social workers.[88]

The organization that today dominates birth control in the United States, the Planned Parenthood Federation, originated in 1942 out of a merger of birth control groups, and is beyond the scope of this article. Nevertheless, it represents the culmination of the tendencies which the professionals introduced in the 1920s and 1930s: removing the focus of birth control education from women's rights to family stability, social unity, and population control. For example, Planned Parenthood continued the efforts of the original birth controllers in promoting sex education, but its content was subtly changed. Planned Parenthood spokespeople avoided the connotation that women might wish to remain childless, affirming motherhood as the main source of women's fulfillment, and arguing merely for the economic and health benefits of small families. They offered a male-centered sex education which perpetuated many existing myths about female sexuality, such as the vaginal orgasm and dangers of promiscuity. Planned Parenthood long clung to a policy of offering birth control services only to married women. That policy in practice supported the prevailing ethic that sex belonged only with marriage; it also supported in effect the double standard, the view that unmarried women who "went all the way" had to "take their chances." Choosing not to challenge conventional norms about women's roles in society—full-time wifehood and motherhood as primary—Planned Parenthood therefore had to argue for birth control in terms of health and population control primarily. And these two themes, as we have seen, were interpreted to the public under the influence of doctors and eugenists. The experts defined good social policy for the public. They held up small families as a model for all people, regardless of other economic and psychologic needs, and without relating family size to the overall quality of life. The planned parenthood/population control merger of the 1950s reflected the experts' sense of their responsibility for offering the small family as a solution for pov-

erty all over the world, with increasing insensitivity to the personal and cultural preferences of other people.

None of these criticisms should obscure the fact that the availability of efficient birth control provided the basis for a radical change in women's possibilities. Lack of control over pregnancy (except through avoiding marriage, which was not an economic or social possibility for most women) and the great burdens of child-raising had represented the single most important factor in women's inequality, probably from the beginning of the species. Placing reproduction under individual control has the potential of making any opportunity available to men open to women also. But the vast majority of women never won these advantages. It is precisely because the liberating potential of birth control for women was so great that the failure of the birth control movement thus far to reach its potential seems regrettable, and is worth analyzing.

Part of the problem lies in the inadequate quantity of birth control services available. But many women do not take advantage of birth control techniques available to them: their problem is social and economic, not merely technologic. For women to desire limiting their pregnancies and to be able to take the responsibility for contraception, they must have a new way of looking at what women should be, a new image of femininity and a new set of actual possibilities that do not require sexual passivity, maternalness, domesticity, self-sacrifice, and the absence of ambition. It was this new sense of womanhood that the birth controllers of the early twentieth century were after. Margaret Sanger believed in 1916 that birth control was revolutionary because it could provide the technologic basis for women to control not only their pregnancies, but their destinies.

Historically, the technology of birth control did not lead, but followed, the social demand for it. Today, too, women have tended to use contraception to the extent that they have other activities that they find preferable to child-raising. The birth control movement was once part of an overall feminist movement, struggling for more opportunities for women in many areas simultaneously, for a total self-determination for women. Lacking that overall movement, birth control has become a part of the

technologic revolution, attempting to create social reform through a single invention, and without the process of liberation that is entailed in a movement of people struggling for their own interests.

Because birth control became removed from a larger social movement, it lost the political content that identified it with the struggle for human liberation. Indeed, one of the problems birth control advocates face today is that many associate birth control with the opposite of liberation—with elitist and racist policies leading even to genocide. There is truth in that belief. Population controllers have used coercion and trickery to impose birth control, often in the form of permanent sterilization, upon Third World peoples such as Puerto Ricans and Indians. Many poor people associate birth control with feminism and disapprove of both. They have experienced feminism as the struggle of privileged women for equality with the men of their privileged classes. It is true that the feminist movement primarily reflected the needs of privileged women in the past; it is also true that the discrimination such women faced, within the birth control movement, for example, paralleled that directed against working-class people. The birth control professionals felt confident that they knew how to arrange the social advancement of less privileged groups, and offered contraception as a panacea. In fact, for women and for all poor people birth control represents a major step forward only when it is combined with campaigns for equality on many fronts.

The struggle for birth control today offers opportunities for those concerned with the welfare of women and of the poor—for those concerned with social equality in general—to change its previously elitist direction. The history of the birth control movement suggests that it is possible to make of it a popular cause that reaches people of all classes if its basic principle is self-determination through increasing the real choices that people have. Legalized abortion that remains out of the price range of most women does not, for example, represent real self-determination. Offering women contraceptives without thorough, female-centered sex education does not represent self-determination. Offering women inadequately tested pills,

and testing those pills on poor and nonwhite women as has been the custom of the drug companies, does not represent self-determination, nor is it likely to make poor people favorably inclined toward birth control as a reform. Similarly, it makes no sense to offer advice or contraceptives without adequate general medical care, or to offer it through disrespectful and condescending doctors. Self-determination must mean a birth control program that is part of an overall program of good medical care, education, respect, and equal opportunity for all women.

NOTES

1. L. Gordon, "Voluntary Motherhood," *Feminist Studies* 1, nos. 3–4 (1972–73): 5–22.
2. This does not mean that contraception was not practiced in the nineteenth century. In fact, there was widespread use of douches, male withdrawal, abortion, and vaginal pessaries to prevent or interrupt pregnancy.
3. C. J. Karier, "Testing for Order and Control," in *Roots of Crisis: American Education in the Twentieth Century*, ed. C. J. Karier, P. Violas, and J. Spring (Chicago: Rand-McNally, 1973), p. 122.
4. H. Goddard, *Psychology of the Normal and Subnormal* (New York: Dodd, Mead, 1919).
5. Karier, "Testing for Order and Control," p. 121.
6. Ibid., p. 122.
7. M. Fishbein, *Medical Follies* (New York: Boni & Liveright, 1925), p. 142.
8. F. McCann, "Presidential Address to League of National Life," *Medical Press and Circular*, November 3, 1926, p. 359.
9. G. Kosmak, in *Bulletin, Lying-In Hospital of the City of New York* (August 1917): 181–92.
10. Ibid.
11. Ibid.
12. D. Kennedy, *Birth Control in America: The Career of Margaret Sanger* (New Haven: Yale University Press, 1970), p. 179.
13. R. L. Dickinson, letter to J. Bentley Squier, November 10, 1925. Dickinson Manuscripts, Countway Library, Harvard University Medical School, Boston.
14. Ibid.

15. Kennedy, *Birth Control in America*, p. 191.
16. Ibid., p. 190; J. Reed, "Birth Control and the Americans: 1830–1970, Part III: Robert L. Dickinson and the Committee on Maternal Health" (Ph.D. diss., Harvard University, 1974), pp. 77–82; L. Lader, *The Margaret Sanger Story* (Garden City, N.Y.: Doubleday, 1955), p. 216.
17. F. M. Vreeland, American Birth Control League files. In "The Process of Reform with Especial Reference to Reform Groups in the Field of Population" (Ph.D. diss., University of Michigan, 1929), p. 280.
18. M. Sanger, letter to J. Noah Slee, February 22, 1925. Sanger Manuscripts, Library of Congress, Washington, D.C.
19. W. N. Wishard, Sr., "Contraception: Are Our County Societies Being Used for the American Birth Control League Propaganda?" *J. Indiana State Med. Assoc.* (May 1929): 187–89.
20. *Proceedings, Sixth International Birth Control Conference*, vol. III (New York: American Birth Control League, 1925), pp. 19–30, 49–60.
21. Vreeland, American Birth Control League files. In "The Process of Reform," p. 280.
22. Kennedy, *Birth Control in America*, pp. 193–96.
23. Mimeographed letter to Voluntary Parenthood League members from President Myra P. Gallert, December 2, 1925. Alice Park Manuscripts, Stanford University Library, Stanford, Cal.
24. M. W. Dennett, *Birth Control Laws* (New York: Frederick H. Hitchcock, 1926), pp. 72–93.
25. A. F. Konikow, "The Doctor's Dilemma in Massachusetts," *Birth Control Review* 15, no. 1 (1931): 21–22.
26. C. C. Jack, in *Birth Control Review* 2, no. 3 (1918): 7–8.
27. C. C. Jack, letter to Charles Birtwell, June 17, 1917. Ames Manuscripts, Sophia Smith Collection, Smith College Library, Northampton, Mass.
28. C. C. Jack, letter to Blanche Ames Ames, January 7, 1918. Ames Manuscripts, Sophia Smith Collection, Smith College Library, Northampton, Mass.
29. Birth Control League of Massachusetts Records, Schlesinger Library, Radcliffe College, Cambridge, Mass.
30. Ibid.
31. Konikow, "The Doctor's Dilemma."
32. Birth Control League of Massachusetts Records, Schlesinger Library, Radcliffe College, Cambridge, Mass.

33. *Boston Post*, July 25, 1916. Quoted in D. McCarrick Geig, "The Birth Control League of Massachusetts" (B.A. thesis, Simmons College, 1973), p. 21.

34. Dennett, *Birth Control Laws*, pp. 72–93.

35. Birth Control and Public Policy, Decision of Judge Harry M. Fisher of the Circuit Court of Cook County, November 23, 1929. Illinois Birth Control League, 1924 (pamphlet).

36. Kennedy, *Birth Control in America*.

37. Ibid., p. 197.

38. M. Sanger, *Autobiography* (New York: W. W. Norton, 1938), pp. 374, 402–8.

39. C. C. Little, letter to Robert L. Dickinson, October 28, 1925. Sanger Manuscripts, Library of Congress, Washington, D.C.

40. Sanger, *Autobiography*, p. 374.

41. D. K. Pickens, *Eugenics and the Progressives* (Nashville: Vanderbilt University Press, 1968), p. 51.

42. Ibid.

43. M. Haller, *Eugenics: Hereditarian Attitudes in American Thought* (New Brunswick, N.J.: Rutgers University Press, 1963), p. 174.

44. I call these assumptions because nothing in the genetic theory that they relied upon, even as it progressed to Mendel's mathematically sophisticated and predictive models, provided any basis for judgment about the relative impact of heredity and environment in producing characteristics such as feeblemindedness, insanity, laziness, and other common eugenic bugaboos.

45. Karier, "Testing for Order and Control," pp. 115–16.

46. P. Popenoe, *The Conservation of the Family* (Baltimore: Williams and Wilkins, 1926), pp. 129–30.

47. M. F. Guyer, *Well-Born. An Introduction to Eugenics* (Indianapolis: Bobbs-Merrill, 1916), pp. 296–98.

48. L. Stoddard, *Revolt Against Civilization: The Menace of the Under Man* (New York: Scribners, 1922), p. 21.

49. Haller, *Eugenics: Hereditarian Attitudes*, p. 55.

50. Fourth Report, Committee on Selective Immigration, American Eugenics Society, June 30, 1928, p. 16. Anita Newcomb McGee Manuscripts, Library of Congress, Washington, D.C.

51. P. Popenoe and R. H. Johnson, *Applied Eugenics* (New York: Macmillan, 1918), pp. 294–97.

52. F. Lorimer, E. Winston, and L. K. Kiser, *Foundations of American Population Policy* (New York: Harper and Brothers, 1940), pp. 12–15.

53. S. H. Halford, "Dysgenic Tendencies of Birth-Control and of the Feminist Movement," in *Population and Birth Control*, ed. Eden and Cedar Paul (New York: Critic and Guide, 1917), p. 238.
54. H. Bergen, "Eugenics and the Social Problem," *Birth Control Review* 4, no. 4 (1920): 5–6, 15–17.
55. E. Paul, "Eugenics and Birth-Control," in *Population and Birth Control*, p. 134.
56. Bergen, "Eugenics and the Social Problem."
57. L. Quessel, "Race Suicide in the United States," in *Population and Birth Control*.
58. Letter of December 20, 1865, from Elizabeth Stanton to Martha Wright, in *Elizabeth Cady Stanton as Revealed in Her Letters, Diary and Reminiscences*, ed. T. Stanton and H. Stanton Blatch (New York: Harper and Brothers, 1922).
59. A. Kraditor, *Ideas of the Woman Suffrage Movement 1890–1920* (New York: Columbia University Press, 1965), ch. 7.
60. M. Sanger, "Why Not Birth Control Clinics in America?" *Birth Control Review* 3, no. 5 (1919): 10–11.
61. M. Sanger, *Woman and the New Race* (New York: Brentano's, 1920), p. 34.
62. M. Sanger, *The Pivot of Civilization* (New York: Brentano's, 1922), pp. 177–78.
63. Stenographic Record of the Proceedings of the First American Birth Control Conference, 1921 (New York: American Birth Control League, 1921), p. 24.
64. "The Necessity for Birth Control." Speech by Margaret Sanger in Oakland, Cal., December 19, 1928. Stenographic record in Sanger Manuscripts, Library of Congress, Washington, D.C.
65. "My Way to Peace." Speech by Margaret Sanger to New History Society, January 17, 1932. Margaret Sanger Manuscripts, Smith College Library, Northampton, Mass.
66. "The Necessity for Birth Control." Speech by Margaret Sanger.
67. *Report of the Fifth International Neo-Malthusian and Birth Control Conference*, ed. R. Pierpont (London: Heinemann, 1922).
68. *Proceedings, Sixth International Birth Control Conference*, vol. III (New York: American Birth Control League, 1925), pp. 19–30, 49–60.
69. P. Popenoe, in *Birth Control Review* 1, no. 3 (1917): 6.
70. W. Thompson, "Race Suicide in the United States," *Birth Control Review* 4, no. 8: 9–10; 4, no. 9: 9–10; 4, no. 10: 10–11; 4, no. 11: 14; 5, no. 1 (1920): 16; 5, no. 2: 9–12; 5, no. 3 (1921): 11–13.

71. "Immigration and Birth Control" (editorial). *Birth Control Review* 7, no. 9 (1923): 219–20.

72. M. Winsor, "The Cost to the State of the Socially Unfit," *Birth Control Review* 7, no. 9 (1923): 222–24.

73. H. Ellis, "Review of Lothrop Stoddard's *The Rising Tide of Color Against White World Supremacy*," *Birth Control Review* 4, no. 10 (1920): 14–16.

74. C. C. Little, "Unnatural Selection and Its Resulting Obligations," *Birth Control Review* 10, no. 8 (1926): 243–44, 257.

75. Kennedy, *Birth Control in America*, p. 119.

76. Vreeland, American Birth Control League Files. In "The Process of Reform," p. 232.

77. Dr. Richard N. Pierson, president; Dr. Woodbridge E. Morris, general director; vice-presidents were Dr. Robert Latou Dickinson, Henry Pratt Fairchild, Frederick C. Holden, Clarence C. Little, and Charles Edward Amory Winslow. Little and Fairchild were eugenists. Winslow was closely associated with Rockefeller family enterprises.

78. Kennedy, *Birth Control in America*, p. 200.

79. K. B. Davis, *Factors in the Sex Life of Twenty-Two Hundred Women* (New York: Harper and Brothers, 1929); L. Terman, *Psychological Factors in Marital Happiness* (New York: McGraw-Hill, 1938); G. V. T. Hamilton, *A Research in Marriage* (New York: A. & C. Boni, 1929).

80. Kennedy, *Birth Control in America*, p. 202.

81. Davis, *Factors in the Sex Life of Twenty-Two Hundred Women*, p. 44.

82. Kennedy, *Birth Control in America*, p. 200.

83. C. H. Robinson, *Seventy Birth Control Clinics* (Baltimore: Williams and Wilkins, 1930), ch. 4.

84. Sanger, *Autobiography*, pp. 374–75.

85. Robinson, *Seventy Birth Control Clinics*, pp. 50–52.

86. F. S. Jaffe and S. Polgar, "Family Planning and Public Policy: Is the 'Culture of Poverty' the New Cop-Out?" in *Readings in Family Planning*, ed. Donald V. McCalister, Victor Thiessen, and Margaret McDermott (St. Louis: C. V. Mosby, 1973), p. 169.

87. H. P. Fairchild, speech. Planned Parenthood Federation of America Manuscripts, Sophia Smith Collection, Smith College Library, Northampton, Mass., p. 169.

88. Linda Gordon, *Woman's Body, Woman's Right* (New York: Grossman/Viking, 1976).

DORIS HAIRE

THE CULTURAL WARPING OF CHILDBIRTH

While Sweden and the Netherlands compete for the honor of having the lowest incidence of infant deaths per one thousand live births, the United States continues to find itself outranked by fourteen other developed countries.[1] A spokesman for the National Foundation March of Dimes recently stated that according to the most recent data, the United States leads all developed countries in the rate of infant deaths due to birth injury and respiratory distress such as postnatal asphyxia and atelectasis. According to the National Association for Retarded Children there are now six million retarded children and adults in the United States with a predicted annual increase of over 100,000 a year. The number of children and adults with behavioral difficulties or perceptual dysfunction resulting from minimal brain damage is an ever growing challenge to society and to the economy.

While it may be easier on the conscience to blame such numbing facts solely on socioeconomic factors and birth defects, recent research makes it evident that obstetrical medication can play a role in our staggering incidence of neurological impairment. It may be convenient to blame our relatively poor infant outcome on a lack of facilities or inadequate government funding, but it is obvious from the research being carried out that we could effect an immediate improvement in infant outcome by changing the pattern of obstetrical care in the United States. It is time that we take a good look at the overall experience of

This essay is a substantially abridged version of a pamphlet available from ICEA Supplies Center, P.O. Box 70258, Seattle, Washington 98107, for $1.20.

185

childbirth in this country and begin to recognize how our culture has warped this experience for the majority of American mothers and their newborn infants.

As an officer of the International Childbirth Education Association, I have visited hundreds of maternity hospitals throughout the world—in Great Britain, Western Europe, Russia, Asia, Australia, New Zealand, the South Pacific, the Americas, and Africa. During my visits I was privileged to observe obstetric techniques and procedures and to interview physicians, professional midwives, and parents in the various countries. My companion on many of my visits was Dorothea Lang, C.N.M. (Certified Nurse-Midwife), Director of Nurse-Midwifery for New York City. Miss Lang's experience as both a nurse-midwife and a former head nurse of the labor and delivery unit of the New York-Cornell Medical Center made her a particularly well-qualified observer and companion. As we traveled from country to country certain patterns of care soon became evident. For one, in those countries that enjoy an incidence of infant mortality and birth trauma significantly lower than that of the United States, highly trained professional midwives are an important source of obstetrical care and family planning services for normal women, whether the births take place in the hospital or in the home. In these countries the expertise of the physician is called upon only when the expectant mother is ill during pregnancy, or when labor or birth is anticipated to be, or is found to be, abnormal. Under this system, the high-risk mother—the one who is most likely to bear an impaired or stillborn child—has a better opportunity to obtain in-depth medical attention than is possible under our existing American system of obstetrical care where the obstetrician is also called upon to play the role of midwife.

Deprivation, birth defects, prematurity, and low birth weight are not unique to the United States. While it is tempting to blame our comparatively high incidence of infant mortality solely on a lack of available prenatal care and on socioeconomic factors, our observations indicate that, comparatively, the prenatal care we offer most clinic patients in the United States is not grossly inferior to that available in other developed countries. Further-

more, the diet and standard of living in many countries which have a lower incidence of infant mortality than ours would be considered inadequate by American standards.

As an example, when one compares the availability of prenatal care, the incidence of premature births, the average diet of various economic groups, and the equipment available to aid in newborn-infant survival in two such diverse countries as the United States and Japan, there are no major differences between the two countries. The differences lie in (a) our frequent use of prenatal and obstetrical medication, (b) our pathologically oriented management of pregnancy, labor, birth, and postpartum, and (c) the predominance of artificial feeding in the United States, in contrast to Japan.

If present statistics follow the trend of recent years, an infant born in the United States is more than four times more likely to die in the first day of life than an infant born in Japan. But a survival of the birth process should not be our singular goal. For every American newborn infant who dies there are likely to be several who are neurologically damaged.

Unfortunately, the American tendency to warp the birth experience, distorting it into a pathological event rather than a physiological one for the normal childbearing woman, is no longer peculiar to just the United States. In my visits to hospitals in various countries I was distressed to find that some physicians, anxious to impress their colleagues with their "Americanized" techniques, have unfortunately adopted many of our obstetrical practices without stopping to question their scientific or social merit.

Few American babies are born today as nature intended them to be.

It is not unlikely that unnecessary alterations in the normal fetal environment may play a role in the incidence of neurological impairment and infant mortality in the United States. Infant resuscitation, other than routine suctioning, is rarely needed in countries such as Sweden, the Netherlands, and Japan, where the skillful psychological management of labor usually precludes the need for obstetrical medication. In contrast, in those Euro-

pean countries, such as Belgium, where the overall pattern of obstetrical care is similar to our own, the incidence of infant mortality also approaches our own.

Obviously there will always be medical indications which dictate the use of various obstetrical procedures, but to apply the following American practices and procedures routinely to the vast majority of mothers who are capable of giving birth without complication is to create added stress which is not in the best interests of either the mother or her newborn infant.

Let us take a close look at some of our common obstetrical practices from early pregnancy to postpartum which have served to warp and distort the childbearing experience in the United States. While not all of the practices below affect infant mortality, it is equally apparent that they do not contribute to the reduction of infant morbidity or mortality and therefore should be reevaluated.

Withholding information on the disadvantages of obstetrical medication. Ignorance of the possible hazards of obstetrical medication appears to encourage the misuse and abuse of obstetrical medication, for in those countries where mothers are not told routinely of the possible disadvantages of obstetrical medication to themselves or to their babies the use of such medication is on the increase.

There is no research or evidence which indicates that mothers will be emotionally damaged if they are advised, prior to birth, that obstetrical medication may be to the disadvantage of their newborn infants.

Requiring all normal women to give birth in the hospital. While ICEA does not encourage home births, there is ample evidence in the Netherlands and in Chicago (Chicago Maternity Center) to demonstrate that normal women who have received adequate prenatal care can safely give birth at home if a proper system is developed for home deliveries. Over half of the mothers in the Netherlands give birth at home with the assistance of a professional midwife and a maternity aide. The comparatively low incidence of infant deaths and birth trauma in the Netherlands, a country of diverse ethnic composition and inter-

marriage, is evidence of the comparative safety of a properly developed home delivery service.

Dutch obstetricians point out that when the labor of a normal woman is unhurried and allowed to progress normally, unexpected emergencies rarely occur. They also point out that the small risk involved in a Dutch home delivery is more than offset by the increased hazards resulting from the use of obstetrical medication and obstetrical tampering which are more likely to occur in a hospital environment, especially in countries where professionals have had little or no exposure to normal labor and birth in a home environment during their training.

Elective induction of labor. The elective induction of labor (where there is no clear medical indication) appears to be an American idiosyncrasy which is frowned upon in other developed countries.

The elective induction of labor has been found almost to double the incidence of fetomaternal transfusion and its attendant hazards.[2] But perhaps the least appreciated problem of elective induction is the fact that the abrupt onset of artificially induced labor tends to make it extremely difficult for even the well-prepared mother to tolerate the discomfort of the intensified contractions without the aid of obstetrical medication. When the onset of labor occurs spontaneously, the normal, gradual increase in contraction length and intensity appears to provoke in the mother an accompanying tolerance for discomfort or pain.

Since the British Perinatal Hazards Study found no increase in perinatal mortality or impairment of learning ability at age seven among full-term infants unless gestation had extended beyond forty-one weeks,[3] there would appear to be no medical justification for subjecting a mother or her baby to the possible hazards of elective induction in order to terminate the pregnancy prior to forty-one weeks' gestation.

Separating the mother from familial support during labor and birth. Research indicates that fear adversely affects uterine motility and blood flow,[4] and yet many American mothers are routinely separated from a family member or close friend at this time of emotional crisis.

In most developed countries, other than the United States and the Eastern European countries, mothers are encouraged to walk about or to sit and chat with a family member or supportive person in what is called an "early labor lounge." This lounge is usually located near but outside the labor-delivery area in order to provide a more relaxed atmosphere during much of labor. The mother is taken to the labor-delivery area to be checked periodically, then allowed to return to the labor lounge for as long as she likes or until her membranes have ruptured.

Confining the normal laboring woman to bed.   In virtually all countries except the United States, a woman in labor is routinely encouraged to walk about during labor for as long as she wishes or until her membranes have ruptured. Such activity is considered to facilitate labor by distracting the mother's attention from the discomfort or pain of her contractions and to encourage a more rapid engagement of the fetal head. In America, where drugs are frequently administered either orally or parenterally to laboring mothers, such ambulation is discouraged—not only for the patient's safety but also to avoid possible legal complications in the event of an accident.

Shaving the birth area.   Research involving 7,600 mothers has demonstrated that the practice of shaving the perineum and pubis does not reduce the incidence of infection. In fact, the incidence of infection was slightly higher among those mothers who were shaved.[5] Yet this procedure, which tends to create apprehension in laboring women, is still carried out routinely in most American hospitals. Clipping the perineal or pudendal hair closely with surgical scissors is far less disturbing to the mother and is less likely to result in infection caused by razor abrasions.

Professional dependence on technology and pharmacological methods of pain relief.   Most of the world's mothers receive little or no drugs during pregnancy, labor, or birth. The constant emotional support provided the laboring woman in other countries by the nurse-midwife, and often by her husband, appears greatly to improve the mother's tolerance for discomfort. In contrast, the American labor room nurse is frequently assigned to look after several women in labor, all or most of whom have had no preparation to cope with the discomfort or pain of childbear-

ing. Under the circumstances, drugs, rather than skillful emotional support, are employed to relieve the mother's apprehension and discomfort (and perhaps to assuage the harried labor attendant's feeling of inadequacy).

Routine Electronic Fetal Monitoring. The wisdom of depending on an experienced nurse using a stethoscope to monitor accurately the effects of obstetrical medication on the well-being of the fetus has been demonstrated by Haverkamp.[6] No one knows the long-term or delayed consequences of ultrasonic fetal monitoring on subsequent human development. The fact that some electronic fetal monitoring devices require that a mother's membranes be ruptured and the the electrode be screwed into the skin of the fetal scalp creates hazards of its own. Current research indicates that obstetrical management which reduces the need for such monitoring is advisable.

Chemical stimulation of labor. Oxytocic agents are frequently administered to American mothers in order to intensify artificially the frequency or the strength of the mother's contractions, as a means of shortening the mother's labor. While chemical stimulation is sometimes medically indicated, often it is undertaken to satisfy the American propensity for efficiency and speed. Hon suggests that the overenthusiastic use of oxytocic stimulants sometimes results in alterations in the normal fetal heart rate.[7] Fields points out that the possible hazards inherent in elective induction are also possible in artificially stimulated labor unless the mother and fetus are carefully monitored.[8]

Shortening the phases of normal labor when there is no sign of fetal distress has not been shown to improve infant outcome. Little is known of the long-term effects of artificially stimulating labor contractions. During a contraction the unborn child normally receives less oxygen. The gradual buildup of intensity, which occurs when the onset of labor is allowed to occur spontaneously and to proceed without chemical stimulation, appears likely to be a protective mechanism that is best left unaltered unless there is a clear medical indication for the artificial stimulation of labor.

Delaying birth until the physician arrives. Because of the increased likelihood of resultant brain damage to the infant the

practice of delaying birth by anesthesia or physical restraint until the physician arrives to deliver the infant is frowned upon in most countries. Yet the practice still occurs occasionally in the United States and in countries where hospital-assigned midwives do not routinely manage the labor and delivery of normal mothers.

Requiring the mother to assume the lithotomy position for birth. There is gathering scientific evidence that the unphysiological lithotomy position (back flat, with knees drawn up and spread wide apart by "stirrups"), which is preferred by most American physicians because it is more convenient for the *accoucheur*, tends to alter the normal fetal environment and obstruct the normal process of childbearing, making spontaneous birth more difficult or impossible.

The lithotomy and dorsal positions tend to:

1. Adversely affect the mother's blood pressure, cardiac return, and pulmonary ventilation.[9]

2. Decrease the normal intensity of the contractions.[10]

3. Inhibit the mother's voluntary efforts to push her baby out spontaneously[11] which, in turn, increases the need for fundal pressure or forceps and increases the traction necessary for a forceps extraction.

4. Inhibit the spontaneous expulsion of the placenta[12] which, in turn, increases the need for cord traction, forced expression, or manual removal of the placenta[13]—procedures which significantly increase the incidence of fetomaternal hemorrhage.[14]

5. Increase the need for episiotomy because of the increased tension on the pelvic floor and the stretching of the perineal tissue.[15]

Australian, Russian, and American research bears out the clinical experience of European physicians and midwives—that when mothers are supported to a semisitting position for birth, with their feet supported by the lower section of the labor-delivery bed, mothers tend to push more effectively, appear to need less pain relief, are more likely to want to be conscious for birth, and are less likely to need an episiotomy.[16]

The increased efficiency of the semisitting position, combined with a minimum use of medication for birth, is evidenced by the

fact that the combined use of both forceps and the vacuum extractor rarely exceeds 4 percent to 5 percent of all births in the Netherlands, as compared to an incidence of 65 percent in many American hospitals. (Cesarean section occurs in approximately 1.5 percent of all Dutch births.)

The routine use of regional or general anesthesia for delivery. In light of the current shortage of qualified anesthetists and anesthesiologists and the frequent scientific papers now being published on the possible hazards resulting from the use of regional and general anesthesia, it would seem prudent to make every effort to prepare the mother physically and mentally to cope with the sensations and discomfort of birth in order to avoid the use of such medicaments. Regional and general anesthesia not only tend adversely to affect fetal environment pharmacologically, which has been discussed previously herein, but their use also increases the need for obstetrical intervention in the normal process of birth, since both types of anesthesia tend to prolong labor.[17] Johnson points out that peridural and spinal anesthesia significantly increase the incidence of midforceps delivery and its attendant hazards.[18] Pudendal block anesthesia not only tends to interfere with the mother's ability effectively to push her baby down the birth canal due to the blocking of the afferent path of the pushing reflex, but also appears to interfere with the mother's normal protective reflexes, thus making "an explosive" birth and perineal damage more likely to occur.

The routine use of forceps for delivery. There is no scientific justification for the routine application of forceps for delivery.[19] The incidence of delivery by forceps and vacuum extractor, combined, rarely rises above 5 percent in countries where mothers actively participate in the births of their babies. In contrast, as mentioned previously, the incidence of forceps extraction frequently rises to as high as 65 percent in some American hospitals.

Routine episiotomy. There is no research or evidence to indicate that routine episiotomy (a surgical incision to enlarge the vaginal orifice) reduces the incidence of pelvic relaxation (structural damage to the pelvic floor musculature) in the mother. Nor is there any research or evidence that routine episiotomy reduces

neurological impairment in the child who has shown no signs of fetal distress or that the procedure helps to maintain subsequent male or female sexual response.

The incidence of pelvic floor relaxation appears to be on the decline throughout the world, even in those countries where episiotomy is still comparatively rare. The contention that the modern washing machine has been more effective in reducing pelvic relaxation among American mothers than has routine episiotomy is given some credence by the fact that in areas of the United States where life is still hard for the woman pelvic relaxation appears in white women who have never borne children.

In developed countries where episiotomy is comparatively rare the physiotherapist is considered an important member of the obstetrical team—before as well as after birth. The physiotherapist is responsible for seeing that each mother begins exercises the day following birth which will help to restore the normal elasticity and tone of the mother's perineal and abdominal muscles. In countries where every effort is made to avoid the need for an episiotomy, interviews with both parents and professionals indicate that an intact perineum which is strengthened by postpartum exercises is more apt to result in both male and female sexual satisfaction than is a perineum that has been incised and reconstructed.

Why then, is there such an emotional attachment among professionals to routine episiotomy? A prominent European professor of obstetrics and gynecology recently made the following comment on the American penchant for routine episiotomy, "Since all the physician can really do to affect the course of childbirth for the 95 percent of mothers who are capable of giving birth without complication is to offer the mother pharmacological relief from discomfort or pain and to perform an episiotomy, there is probably an unconscious tendency for many professionals to see these practices as indispensable."

Interviews with obstetrician-gynecologists in many countries indicate that they tend to agree that a superficial, first-degree tear is less traumatic to the perineal tissue than an incision which requires several sutures for reconstruction. There is no research which would indicate otherwise.

Early clamping or "milking" of the umbilical cord. Several years ago De Marsh stated that the placental blood normally belongs to the infant and his or her failure to get this blood is equivalent to submitting him or her to a rather severe hemorrhage. Despite the fact that placental transfusion normally occurs in every corner of the world without adverse consequences, there is still a great effort in the United States and Canada to deprecate the practice. One must read the literature carefully to find that placental transfusion has not been demonstrated to increase the incidence of morbidity or mortality in the placentally transfused infant.[20]

Delaying the first breast-feeding. The common American practice of routinely delaying the time of the first breast-feeding has not been shown to be in the best interest of either the conscious mother or her newborn infant. Clinical experience with the early feeding of newborn infants has shown this practice to be safe.[21] If the mother feels well enough and the infant is capable of suckling while they are still in the delivery room then it would seem more cautious, in the event of tracheoesophageal abnormality, to permit the infant to suckle for the first time under the watchful eye of the physician or nurse-midwife rather than delay the feeding for several hours when the expertise of the professional may not be immediately available.

In light of the many protective antibodies contained in colostrum it would seem likely that the earlier the infant's intake of species specific colostrum, the sooner the antibodies can be accrued by the infant.

Offering water and formula to the breast-fed newborn infant. The common American practice of giving water or formula to a newborn infant prior to the first breast-feeding or as a supplement during the first days of life has not been shown to be in the best interests of the infant. There are now indications that these practices may, in fact, be harmful. Glucose water, once the standby in every American hospital, has now been designated a potential hazard if aspirated by the newborn infant, yet it is still used in many American hospitals.

Restricting newborn infants to a four-hour feeding schedule and withholding nightime feedings. Although widely spaced

infant feedings may be more convenient for hospital personnel, the practice of feeding a newborn infant only every four
hours and not permitting the infant to breast-feed at all during
the night cannot be justified on any scientific grounds. Such a
regimen restricts the suckling stimulation necessary to bring
about the normally rapid onset and adequate production of the
mother's milk. In countries where custom permits the infant to
suckle immediately after birth and on demand from that time,
first-time mothers frequently begin to produce breast milk for
their babies within twenty-four hours after birth. In contrast, in
countries where hospital routines prevent normal demand-
feeding from birth, mothers frequently do not produce breast
milk for their babies until the third day following birth.

Overdistention of the breast or engorgement is a hospital-
acquired condition which does not occur to any comparable
degree in cultures where mothers are permitted to breast-feed
their babies on demand from birth.[22]

Preventing early father-child contact. Permitting fathers to
hold their newborn infants immediately following birth and during the postpartum hospital stay has not been shown by research
or clinical experience to increase the incidence of infection
among newborns, even when those infants are returned to a
regular or central nursery. Yet only in the Eastern European
countries is the father permitted less involvement in the immediate postpartum period than in the United States.

Research has consistently confirmed the fact that the greatest
sources of infection to the newborn infant are the nursery and
nursery personnel.[23] One has only to observe a mother holding
her newborn infant against her bathrobe, which has probably
been exposed to abundant hospital-borne bacteria, to realize the
fallacy of preventing a father from holding his baby during the
hospital stay.

*Restricting intermittent rooming-in to specific room require-
ments.* Throughout the world great effort is made to keep
mothers and babies together in the hospital, no matter how
inconvenient the accommodations. There is no research or evidence which indicates that intermittent rooming-in should be
restricted to private rooms or to rooms which have a sink, or

which provide at least eighty square feet for mother and baby. Such requirements are based on conjecture and not on controlled evaluation.

Restricting sibling visitation. The common American practice of prohibiting toddlers and children from visiting their mothers during the hospital stay is an emotional hardship on both the mothers and their children and is unsupported by scientific research or evidence. Experience in other countries and in several hospitals here in the United States suggests that where sibling visitation is permitted, a short explanation as to the importance of not bringing suspect illnesses into the hospital seems to be effective in controlling infection.

SUMMARY

As mentioned previously, most of the practices discussed above have developed not from a lack of concern for the well-being of the mother and baby but from a lack of awareness as to the problems which can arise from each progressive digression from the normal childbearing experience. Like a snowball rolling down hill, as one unphysiological practice is employed, for one reason or another, another frequently becomes necessary to counteract some of the disadvantages, large or small, inherent in the previous procedure.

The higher incidence of fetal, neonatal, and maternal deaths occurring in our large urban hospitals, as opposed to our smaller community hospitals,[24] is undoubtedly due, in part, to the greater proportion of high-risk mothers in the urban areas. But we in the United States must stop looking for scapegoats and face up to the fact that by individualizing the care offered to maternity patients, much can be done immediately to improve infant outcome without the slightest outlay of capital.

There is currently an increasing emphasis on consolidating maternity facilities. However, we in ICEA do not see the consolidation of community obstetrical facilities as being always in the best interest of the vast majority of mothers who are capable of giving birth without complications. There should, of course, be centers where those mothers who have had no prenatal care or

who are anticipated to be obstetrical risks can be properly cared for. But to insist that every healthy mother must go to a major maternity facility which is unnecessary for her needs and inconvenient for her family, and where she is very apt to be "lost in the crowd," will only spur the growing trend in the United States toward professionally unattended home births.

Throughout the United States the current inclination of many expectant parents is to seek out, to "shop around" for the type of physician and hospital they feel they need in order to have the type of childbearing experience they want. They not only want a doctor who will support them in their efforts to have a prepared, natural birth, with a minimum of or no medication; they also want a hospital which offers education for childbearing and a supportive family-centered atmosphere. These expectant mothers appreciate the availability of such facilities as an early labor lounge, a dual purpose labor-delivery room, a mother-baby recovery room, and a children's visiting room if they have older children. But most of all they want a supportive atmosphere in which they can share the childbearing experience to the extent that they desire, and one which makes an effort to meet the individual needs of the mother, the father, and their newborn baby as they form their family bonds during the hospital stay.

NOTES

1. H. Chase, "Ranking Countries by Infant Mortality Rates," *Public Health Reports* 84 (1969): 19–27; M. Wegman, "Annual Summary of Vital Statistics—1969," *Pediatrics* 47 (1971): 461–64.
2. A. Beer, "Fetal Erythrocytes in Maternal Circulation of 155 Rh-Negative Women," *Obstet. & Gynec.* 34 (1969): 143–50.
3. N. Butler, "A National Long-Term Study of Perinatal Hazards," Sixth World Congress of the Federation of International Gynecology & Obstetrics, 1970.
4. J. Kelly, "Effect of Fear Upon Uterine Motility," *Am. J. Obstet. & Gynec.* 83 (1962): 576–81.
5. R. Burchell, "Predelivery Removal of Pubic Hair," *Obstet. & Gynec.* 24 (1964): 272–73; H. Kantor et al., "Value of Shaving the Pudendal-Perineal Area in Delivery Preparation," *Obstet. & Gynec.* 25 (1965): 509–12.
6. Haverkamp, A. D., Thompson, H. E., McFee, J. G. et al., "The

Evaluation of Continuous Fetal-Heart Monitoring for High Risk Pregnancies." *Am. J. Obstet. & Gynec.* 125, no. 3(June 1, 1926): 310–20.

7. E. Hon, "Direct Monitoring of the Fetal Heart," *Hospital Practice* (September 1970): 91–97.

8. H. Fields, "Complications of Elective Induction," *Obstet. & Gynec.* 15 (1960): 476–80; H. Fields, "Induction of Labor: Methods, Hazards, Complications, and Contraindications," *Hospital Topics* (December 1968): 63–68.

9. C. Flowers, *Obstetric Analgesia and Anesthesia* (New York: Hoeber, Harper & Row, 1967); L. S. James, "The Effects of Pain Relief for Labor and Delivery on the Fetus and Newborn," *Anesthesiology* 21 (1960): 405–30; A. Blankfield, "The Optimum Position for Childbirth," *Med. J. Australia* 2 (1965): 666–68.

10. Blankfield, "The Optimum Position for Childbirth"; F. H. Howard, "Delivery in the Physiologic Position," *Obstet. & Gynec.* 11 (1958): 318–22; I. Gritsiuk, "Position in Labor," *Ob-Gyn Observer* (September 1968).

11. Blankfield, "The Optimum Position for Childbirth"; Howard, "Delivery in the Physiologic Position"; N. Newton and M. Newton, "The Propped Position for the Second Stage of Labor," *Obstet. & Gynec.* 15 (1960): 28–34.

12. Newton and Newton, "The Propped Position for the Second Stage of Labor."

13. M. Botha, "The Management of the Umbilical Cord in Labour," *S. Afr. J. Obstet.* 6, no. 2 (1968): 30–33.

14. Beer, "Fetal Erythrocytes in Maternal Circulation of 155 Rh-Negative Women."

15. Blankfield, "The Optimum Position for Childbirth."

16. Ibid.; Newton and Newton, "The Propped Position for the Second Stage of Labor."

17. L. Hellman and J. Pritchard, *Williams Obstetrics*, 14th ed. (New York: Appleton-Century-Crofts, 1971).

18. W. Johnson, "Regionals Can Prolong Labor," *Medical World News*, October 15, 1971.

19. Butler, "A National Long-Term Study of Perinatal Hazards."

20. S. Saigal et al., "Placental Transfusion and Hyperbilirubinemia in the Premature," *Pediatrics* 49 (1972): 406–19.

21. H. Eppink, "Time of Initial Breast Feeding Surveyed in Michigan Hospitals," *Hospital Topics* (June 1968): 116–17.

22. M. Newton and N. Newton, "Postpartum Engorgement of the Breast," *Am. J. Obstet. & Gynec.* 61 (1951): 664–67.

23. H. Gezon et al., "Some Controversial Aspects in the Epidemiology

of Hospital Nursery Staphylococcal Infections," *Amer. J. of Public Health* 50 (1960): 473–84; R. Ravenholt and G. LaVeck, "Staphylococcal Disease—An Obstetric, Pediatric & Community Problem," *Amer. J. of Public Health* 46 (1956): 1287–96.

24. E. Bishop, "The National Study of Maternity Care," *Obstet. & Gynec.* (1971): 745–50.

MARY C. HOWELL
PEDIATRICIANS AND MOTHERS

I would like to share with you an informal content analysis of the written wisdom of pediatricians, expressed in materials designed for teaching, about mothers specifically and women and parents in general. I have reviewed recent editions of two major pediatric texts;[1] I have also looked at the 1974 and 1975 issues of the *Pediatric News*, a newsletter that summarizes presentations at professional meetings of interest to pediatricians.[2] What I have to present is a compendium of horrors. I have made no effort to weigh "bad" attitudes against "good." There are, of course, pediatricians—both practitioners and teachers—who are decent, modest, and respectful. But the very existence of the statements that I have collected is, for me, a source of dismay. It is plain that learning or retaining the kinds of attitudes that enable a pediatrician to provide supportive service to children *in the context of their families* is an uphill fight. Furthermore, much of the attitudinal distortion that I will present here is subtle and quietly reinforces attitudes and assumptions that are already widely prevalent in our society at large, and thus is doubly effective in its consequences.

To start with, you must understand that pediatricians like to see themselves as rescuing children from those who would harm them—*especially parents*. One of the texts begins, "This book is dedicated to the health of children throughout the world, particularly those who are the innocent victims of ignorance and superstition, hunger and poverty, disease and overpopulation."[3] This advertisement shows someone's conception of a pediatrician's ideal self-image: a knight-in-armor, idolized by a Lolita-like child.

Add to this the pervasive disparagement of women—a sex-based stereotyping that is, if anything, more acceptable in the men's locker-room atmosphere of medical education than elsewhere in our society.[4] I assume that most of you are already familiar with attitudes toward women as presented in medical-school teaching. Let me just quote from a report about a presentation on adolescent sexuality:

> Promiscuous, psychiatrically disturbed adolescent girls present the physician with a dilemma of whether to prescribe contraceptives. . . . If the . . . [doctor] prescribes contraceptives, he encourages her pathologic promiscuity. . . . Refusing to prescribe contraceptives . . . however, does not guarantee that she will benefit from psychiatric therapy. No psychiatric therapy can compete with her "sexual version of collecting scalps," which combines aggression with the need to be cuddled. . . . What the adolescent girl who appears to "collect penises" really wants is cuddling. . . . Because the clinging 16-year-old girl may make the younger boy feel trapped, he may deliberately stop using contraceptives in order to get her pregnant. To impregnate the clinging girl is a palpable way of his getting back at her.[5]

Clearly, for this representative of the medical profession, women are dangerous, despised, and to be put down. It is no wonder, then, that women, including mothers, are often objects of disrespect in the eyes of pediatricians.

There are two ways in which this disrespect is manifest in attitudes and behavior. First is the blaming of mothers for their children's health problems, and the parallel mechanism of inducing guilt in women—who are already bombarded by the message that the goodness and well-being of their children will be the measure of their own competence and adequacy. Second, pediatricians oppress mothers by disparaging, if not ignoring, the central and essential contributions made by mothers to promote, maintain, restore, and protect the health of their children. Mothers are, in fact, the primary providers of health care for children, although this is rarely acknowledged. So if something goes wrong with our children's health, we mothers are likely to be blamed; if all goes well, we are rarely credited.

I must say a word about "mothers" and "parents." I am gener-

ally very much opposed to the assumption that only mothers take care of children; in fact, I squirm to read in pediatric texts that all parents are referred to as "she," and all children as "he." (When a parent is referred to as "he" it is usually in a situation of privilege. In a discussion of the rights of parents: "There is also the idea that the parent is entitled to some fun of his own. . . . [We must recognize the need for] the separation of parent and child periodically while the former has some fun of his own."[6] And in a discussion of the ethics of genetic manipulations: "Should the parent be allowed to choose the sex of his child?"[7]) But despite the growing number of U.S. families in which mothers and fathers *both* share the responsibilities of child care, in fact in our society at the present time most child care is still done by mothers, and is pretty much a solo responsibility. So let us acknowledge that fathers who take care of children are also discriminated against in the offices of pediatricians—by the assumption that no self-respecting man could understand, care about, and take part in the day-to-day nurture of his daughters and sons. And then let us focus on the difficulties that mothers face in getting the health-related information and advice needed to safeguard our children.

First, let us look at guilt and blaming. It is not enough, apparently, that our very worth is at stake in our children's health and happiness. A recent article goes one better (or worse, as the case may be): it proposes that if a preschool child shows unexplained developmental delay, this may be taken as *evidence* of occult, previously unrecognized neurosis or emotional disorder in the mother.[8] In other words, if your child is not as advanced as the judging doctor would expect, that judgment proves that you must be crazy.

What about the children of employed mothers? For starters, there is no listing in the index of either text for maternal employment, despite the fact that over half of U.S. mothers of children six to eighteen, and over a third of mothers of children under six, are now in paid employment. I could find only three mentions of maternal employment in one of the texts; two are in the discussion of marasmus—severe protein malnutrition in infants—and imply that maternal employment, and consequent early weaning, are a frequent and primary *cause* of marasmus.[9]

The third mention occurs in the chapter on "The Abdomen and the Gastrointestinal Tract," under the heading "Constipation":

> Another group of children has been characterized as having the "pot-refusal retention syndrome." These children actively refuse to use the pot and tenaciously retain feces. Fecal soiling is common. They may be found with legs crossed, hiding behind furniture, fiercely resisting the reflex mechanisms of their lower bowels. Abdominal distention and palpable fecal masses are commonly found. Punitive parental attitudes are often associated with the early training of these children; one can often elicit a history of broken homes, working mothers, and emotional illnesses in the family background.[10]

Mothers are variously blamed when their children become ill: for bothering the doctor too often, for not having brought the child in early enough, for being unduly alarmed, for not having recognized signs and symptoms of "real" illness. One advertisement in a pediatric journal recommends long-acting injectable penicillin *because mothers can not be trusted* to give oral medication. As a mother, I am the first to agree that it is difficult to remember three doses a day for ten days, and that a single injection of an antibiotic is a convenient treatment for child and parent alike. But I refuse to accept a judgment of moral turpitude for what is just a very human characteristic. I wonder how many male pediatricians have actually given thirty oral penicillin doses to a child?

As another example of the blaming of mothers for their children's health problems, I cite a report on a discussion about the masculinizing effects on female infants of hormones ingested by pregnant women, in which this explanation is given:

> Many women who become pregnant will deny their condition and take birth control pills throughout the pregnancy. As a result, their infants may have the female virilization syndrome.[11]

Mothers are also blamed for incestuous sexual relations between fathers and daughters:

> Father-daughter incest often takes place with the knowledge and tacit consent of the mothers involved. Such mothers are all too happy to let their daughters fulfill their sexual obligations to their

husbands. They often arrange their schedules so that they work nights, leaving the daughter and father ample opportunity for sexual encounters. . . . Even if the mother disapproves, she is often reluctant to report incest to the police out of shame or fear that the husband will be jailed and companionship or income will be lost.[12]

And guess who has been responsible for the bacterial diarrheas of infants? You guessed—mothers! In a discussion indicating disbelief that there might be any special disease-preventing properties in breast milk, a report points out that most studies that demonstrated a lower incidence of dangerous bacterial diarrheas in breast-fed infants were done before prepared artificial infant formulas were readily available:

> In the days when "formula making" was popular . . . it was a common practice for mothers to add a carbohydrate to the formula, which they measured by leveling off a tablespoon with their finger. High *E. coli* counts followed.[13]

Finally, there is the tragic tale of the pediatric prescription for solo mother-only responsibility for preschool child care—a subject too enormous to deal with adequately here. Let me just quote from two articles in one recent issue of *Pediatric News*. One pediatrician urges that infants not be snatched away from their mothers immediately after delivery—a worthy crusade. But he argues that this change in delivery-room practice should be done in order "to lock the mother and baby to each other emotionally."[14] One test of whether this desired outcome is achieved is seen when the infant is one month old—mothers are then expected to be "reluctant to leave their babies in someone else's care."[15] The contrasting article, in the same issue, is about behavior problems in children:

> When first-day-of-school jitters becomes vomiting every morning for weeks . . . it generally indicates a pathologically intense, symbolic love-hate relationship between child and mother. . . . The separation/individuation process was not completed in infancy, and the mother and child are "not yet separate human beings."[16]

It seems to me that if pediatricians push mothers into that locked-in state, they must themselves take some responsibility for the outcome five years later. (As someone who cares intensely about

children *and* mothers, I am increasingly nervous about two topics currently in vogue: child abuse and children's rights. I fear that they can be disguised, and apparently well-meaning rubrics designed literally to lock mothers to children in a relationship that is less than optimal for both.)

The second kind of disparagement of mothers overlooks or ignores mothers' major responsibility for children's health. A commonplace complaint of pediatricians about their work is that "the children are great, but oh, those mothers!" Ideally, at least for some pediatricians, a mother transports the child to the office, speaks only when spoken to—and she had better have on the tip of her tongue the information that the doctor needs to diagnose the child's problem; she carries out the doctor's orders as a docile and self-effacing nurse should, and she sees that the bills are paid.

In fact, mothers carry out the major part of child health care. We promote good health by providing—against odds, I might say—the best nutrition that we can procure. We promote health by encouraging physical exercise—by our own example—in the games we play with our children, and by applauding their participation in their games with others.

By far the great majority of childhood illnesses are cared for at home, by parents, with no recourse to health professionals. We are diagnosticians, noting the early signs of an illness and its progression, and deciding, on each occasion, whether expert assessment and advice are needed. We are therapists, providing vaporizers and Vicks and peppermint tea and chicken soup, not to mention support and guidance for our children's heartbreaks and fears and worries. We decide when an illness is over, and prescribe the sequence of the return to regular activities.

And finally, we provide health care as we try to protect our children from the undue—and I think unnecessary—hazards of living in this society: automobile accidents; machinery that entangles and maims; the poisons of lead paint, gasoline-exhaust polluted earth, and household cleanser; and the dangerous toys advertised on TV and sold in stores. No one else is much concerned with the protection of our children against these unreasonable and often hidden hazards, and we work against great odds.

In all of these functions, we mothers need access to experts for information and guidance. Pediatricians, unfortunately, are generally engrossed with rare and exotic diseases; they are neither very interested nor even very well informed in the kinds of knowledge that we parents need to supplement the care that we give our children. Our poor showing among so-called developed nations with regard to infant mortality is a national disgrace. In 1972, the United States ranked fifteenth, with a rate of 18.5 deaths per 1,000 live births. [17] Socioeconomic status of the mother appears to be the strongest predictor of perinatal disease and death—that is, the babies of poor mothers are especially in danger. Even more clearly, calorie- and protein-deficient maternal diets predictably result in infants with lower birth weights and perhaps even with a reduced number of brain cells. [18] Despite these known problems, in 1974 less than 10 percent of National Institutes of Health (tax) funds for research related to maternal and child health were invested in the three major areas of child health hazards *combined*—i.e., malnutrition, accidents, and environmental poisoning. [19]

As an example of the way that pediatric texts deal with questions such as these, consider the problem of malnutrition in children. In one of those pediatric texts the authors manage to discuss the entire problem of malnutrition without ever mentioning poverty—which I believe constitutes a tour de force of misunderstanding. [20] There is only a passing reference to the increase in malnutrition among children "in areas with insufficient food." Causes of malnutrition of concern to pediatricians learning from this text are poor parent-child relations (especially parental "overanxiety about eating habits"), too much TV-watching, and too many candy bars between meals. At another place in the same text the authors note that because infants must depend on others to bring food to them (that is, they cannot provide food for themselves), "nutritional deficiencies [at this stage] are thus particularly likely to be the *fault* of the person who designs the diet or feeds the infant [emphasis added]." [21]

Further, young pediatricians are taught the following: because the fetus is an efficient parasite, draining the pregnant mother's body of nutriments when her own diet is inadequate, and because

on the other hand the nutritional quality of breast milk is directly dependent on maternal diet, the good doctors who teach pediatrics conclude that "the diet of the lactating mother is probably more critical than that of the pregnant woman."[22] I read that to mean that the authors are relatively unconcerned about poverty, starvation, malnutrition, and poorly balanced diets in adult women, unless the women are breast-feeding.

I will close with a pair of contrasting quotations: the first is from a report, given at the annual meeting of the American Public Health Association, on children and mothers in rural Appalachia:

> Mothers who neglect their children tend to have pervasive severe personality immaturity and social inadequacy and have probably failed at many of life's demands. . . . They reacted to frustration with either temper tantrums, demands for help, or passive resignation. They rarely expressed their ideas or feelings about anything. Group therapy for these women is not recommended. They were so infantile that they could not or would not tolerate the social sharing, suppression of egocentric gratification or the pressure for verbal communication required for group participation [presumably, with this hostile male academic professional as group leader].[23]

It does not make me very comfortable to admit membership in a profession in which at least some members argue that women should be forced to bear children they do not want (for many pediatricians are strongly opposed to abortion), fail to exert any effort to provide mothers with the means and supports that they must have to care for their children (for only a few pediatricians are active in promoting people-oriented social change), and then invent endless new ways to blame mothers for their children's misfortunes (as this paper illustrates). I am happy, however, to conclude with a poem about how mothers feel about feeding and taking care of children. I like to think that Susan Griffin, the author, was one of the mothers in that study:

> I like to think of Harriet Tubman.
> Harriet Tubman who carried a revolver,
> who had a scar on her head from a rock thrown
> by a slave-master (because she
> talked back), and who
> had a ransom on her head

of thousands of dollars and who
was never caught, and who
had no use for the law
when the law was wrong,
who defied the law. I like
to think of her.
I like to think of her especially
when I think of the problem of
feeding children.

The legal answer
to the problem of feeding children
is ten free lunches every month,
being equal, in the child's real life,
to eating lunch every other day.
Monday but not Tuesday.
I like to think of the President
eating lunch Monday, but not
Tuesday.
And when I think of the President
and the law, and the problem of
feeding children, I like to
think of Harriet Tubman
and her revolver.

And then sometimes
I think of the President
and other men,
men who practice the law,
who revere the law,
who enforce the law
who live behind
and operate through
and feed themselves
at the expense of
starving children
because of the law,
men who sit in paneled offices
and think about vacations
and tell women
whose care it is
to feed children

not to be hysterical
not to be hysterical as in the word
hysterikos, the greek for
womb suffering,
not to suffer in their
wombs,
not to care,
not to bother the men
because they want to think
of other things
and do not want
to take the women seriously.
I want them
to take women seriously.
I want them to think about Harriet Tubman,
and remember,
remember she was beat by a white man
and she lived
and she lived to redress her grievances,
and she lived in swamps
and wore the clothes of a man
bringing hundreds of fugitives from
slavery, and was never caught,
and led an army,
and won a battle,
and defied the laws
because the laws were wrong, I want men
to take us seriously.
I am tired wanting them to think
about right and wrong.
I want them to fear.
I want them to feel fear now
as I have felt suffering in the womb, and
I want them
to know
that there is always a time
there is always a time to make right
what is wrong,
there is always a time
for retribution
and that time
is beginning.[24]

NOTES

1. *Textbook of Pediatrics*, ed. W. Nelson, V. Vaughan, and R. McKay, 9th ed. (Philadelphia: W. B. Saunders, 1969); *Pediatrics*, ed. M. Ziai, C. Janeway, and R. Cooke (Boston, Little, Brown, 1969).
2. *Pediatric News* (Washington, D.C.: World Medical Reports, Inc.).
3. Ziai, Janeway, and Cooke, *Pediatrics*, dedication page.
4. M. A. Campbell, *"Why Would a Girl Go Into Medicine?" Medical Education in the United States: A Guide for Women* (Old Westbury, N.Y.: The Feminist Press, 1973).
5. *Pediatric News* 8, no. 4 (1974): 5.
6. *Pediatric News* 8, no. 1 (1974): 51.
7. *Pediatric News* 9, no. 4 (1975): 3.
8. *Pediatric News* 8, no. 3 (1974): 3.
9. Ziai, Janeway, and Cooke, *Pediatrics*, pp. 181, 187.
10. Ibid., p. 378.
11. *Pediatric News* 8, no. 3 (1974): 6.
12. *Pediatric News* 9, no. 3 (1975): 3.
13. *Pediatric News* 9, no. 4 (1975): 31.
14. *Pediatric News* 9, no. 4 (1975): 2.
15. *Pediatric News* 9, no. 3 (1975): 2.
16. *Pediatric News* 9, no. 4 (1975): 67.
17. D. Haire, *The Cultural Warping of Childbirth* (Seattle: International Childbirth Education Association, 1972).
18. *Pediatric News* 7, no. 10 (1974): 15.
19. M. Howell, *Helping Ourselves* (Boston: Beacon Press, 1975).
20. Nelson, Vaughan, and McKay, *Textbook of Pediatrics*, pp. 164–65.
21. Ibid., p. 7.
22. Ziai, Janeway, and Cooke, *Pediatrics*, p. 165.
23. *Pediatric News* 8, no. 1 (1974): 23.
24. S. Griffin, "I Like to Think of Harriet Tubman," in *No More Masks!*, ed. F. Howe and E. Bass (New York: Doubleday Anchor, 1973), pp. 307–9.

DIANA SCULLY AND PAULINE BART

A FUNNY THING HAPPENED ON THE WAY TO THE ORIFICE: WOMEN IN GYNECOLOGY TEXTBOOKS[1]

Feeble and sensitive at birth, and destined by nature to give us existence and to preserve us afterwards by means of her tender and watchful care, woman, the most faithful companion of man, may be regarded as the very complement of the benefits bestowed upon us by the Divine Being: as an object fitted to excite our highest interest and presenting to the philosopher, as well as to the physician, a vast field of contemplation.

Whereas before puberty she existed but for herself alone, when all her charms are in full bloom, she now belongs to the entire species which she is destined to perpetuate by bearing almost all the burden of reproduction.[2]

These words, although written in 1845 in Victorian rhetoric (by gynecologist Dr. Lésère Colombat and translated by Dr. Charles Meigs) illustrate the rationale which has guided the specialty of gynecology and remained almost unchanged to the present day. Man belongs to himself alone, but Woman belongs to Mankind. The vagina is merely a receptacle for the male seed. The coupling, one hopes, will result in impregnation, thus allowing the woman to fulfill her raison d'être—to nurture and maintain, to please and to serve her men and mankind.

However, this quotation makes no mention of frigidity, a subject which occupies much space in later texts. The distinction is made instead between the normal woman of frivolous, romantic emotions and the nymphomaniac who is debased by seeking and enjoying sexual encounters. This reflects the nineteenth-century tenet that women of firm morals did not enjoy sex. It was for them a duty to their husbands and a necessity for motherhood.

Hence the Victorian dictum describing the appropriate role for women in intercourse was, "Ladies do not move."

However, this sentimentalized portrayal of women does not mean that women were esteemed and valued by their physicians. In 1848 Dr. Meigs, discussing vaginal examinations, told a class of medical students, "I am bound to say that it will be your painful, even your distressing, duty, to *condescend* to the task of making such explorations" [emphasis added].[3]

On the East and West coasts the pronunciation is O-B-G-Y-N. In the great heartland of America it is OB-Gyne. But the variation we found was primarily limited to the *pronunciation* of the specialty.[4] For when we examined gynecology books over time, ranging from the pre-Kinsey era through the allegedly revolutionary post-Masters-and-Johnson decade, one factor remained constant: anatomy is destiny. Woman is put on this earth to be fruitful and multiply. Her maternal instinct defines her being, unless of course she is "immature" or "neurotic." She is considered a cranky child with a uterus. Gynecology is a specialty practiced (some say perpetrated) on women by men and for men.

THEORY: HYPOTHESES

The data that we will present can be most fruitfully interpreted when set in the framework of the sociology of knowledge, the analytic tool available for demonstrating the relationship between substructure and superstructure, between interest and ideology, between existential (environmental) factors and the production and interpretation of ideas—whether they be constitutions, theologies, reconstructed histories, or social and behavioral sciences. Since sexism—the taking for granted of society organized in the interest of males and viewed from a male perspective—is ideology, we use the sociology of knowledge for this work.

The basic question to be asked when confronted with a theory is: "Whose interest is this theory in?" The perspective of the sociology of knowledge reveals that gynecology is just another of the forces committed to the maintenance of traditional sex-role stereotypes, in the interest of men and from a male perspective. Thus Taylor notes that there has been since the earliest written

record a tendency for men to explain emotional and hysterical behavior in women as related to the female reproductive tract.[5] There were three Greek words meaning womb, and one Roman word, uterus. The term describing an *emotional state* caused by a derangement or malfunction of the womb was "hysterikas," derived from hystera, one of the three Greek words. Taylor points out:

> It seems of some significance that with the choice of several roots, the one with the additional emotional overlay should survive as our medical word to indicate removal of this organ, hysterectomy. The word hysterectomy has been part of the medical vocabulary for generations. Although the uterus has nothing to do with hysteria, the term hysterectomy persists. Its persistence is significant because accuracy should dictate substitution of the word uterectomy.[6]

There is a growing literature detailing the emphasis on traditional sex roles found in works ranging from children's story and school books through college history and sociology texts and academic disciplines.[7] The work that we are presenting will, we hope, add to this literature.

Gynecology and obstetrics are overwhelmingly a male specialty (6.8 percent female practitioners). The male gynecologist is socialized first as a male and second as a doctor, the latter by the most powerful and elite profession, medicine. As a gynecologist, he is the official and legitimate specialist on women—their personality adjustment, their needs and values, as well as the illnesses associated with the reproductive tract.[8] He wields great power vis-à-vis women seeking to understand their bodies and themselves, particularly their sexuality. As the official expert on women, the gynecologist is in a privileged position to define what is "normal femininity" and "normal sexuality." In this, gynecology textbooks are the official rule books, and we have learned that they perpetuate sexism.[9]

It is our thesis that (1) although some of the Victorian sexual prohibitions and stereotypes have been removed from the rules, new, more sophisticated, and equally repressive ones have taken their place; and (2) the underlying imagery of woman's purpose and place has changed little in 125 years. Women are still de-

picted as primarily put on earth for reproduction and homemaking. These texts continually define female sexuality as inferior to male sexuality, insist that "aggressive" behavior in women is abnormal, and maintain that it is inherent in the female essence to submit to the male. At worst they are hostile and at best paternalistic. One need read only a few of these texts to observe that the authors are primarily concerned with their patients' husbands rather than with their patients. They consider the sick female, the female who neither enjoys coitus nor "innocently simulates" such enjoyment,[10] the female who cannot or will not have children, as a burden and a bother to her man. Moreover, according to a 1968 text,

> If like all human beings, he [the gynecologist] is made in the image
> of the Almighty, and if he is kind, then his kindness and concern for
> this patient may provide her with a glimpse of God's image.[11]

METHOD

The data presented in this paper are the result of content analyses that we completed on twenty-eight gynecology textbooks. Complete lists of texts and authors were obtained from the Index Catalog of the Library of the Surgeon General's Office, National Library of Medicine. In most cases, the texts used were restricted to major volumes published in the United States. Those included in the study represent approximately 80 percent of the authors active in the field of textbook writing since 1943. Part of our interest centered on ascertaining the extent to which the findings of Kinsey and Masters and Johnson, experts on human sexuality, were reflected in gynecology texts. Therefore the research was constructed according to three historical periods: pre-Kinsey, 1943–1952, four texts read; post-Kinsey but pre-Masters-and-Johnson, 1953–1962, nine texts read; and post-Masters-and-Johnson, 1963–1972, fifteen texts read. The earlier periods represent proportionately fewer volumes because major writers periodically update their work, in which case the most recent edition was used.

First we looked for chapters on relevant areas such as premari-

tal examination, marriage counseling, female hygiene, and sexual adjustment. In addition, we searched the indices under such terms as "sex," "frigid," "menstrual problem," and "abortion." In addition, we looked at any chapter referring to psychological factors. Because the format of the books varied and because this study is in the context of discovery rather than verification, a more rigid approach would have been less useful.

THE PERIOD, 1943–1953

In this period, which is prior to the work of Kinsey and Masters and Johnson, female sexuality is almost a complete mystery. However, gynecologists were convinced on several points: (1) the sexual experience of the female was less important, less intense, and less pleasurable than that of the male; (2) the majority of females never experienced orgasm due to their own fundamental inability to do so; and (3) the "true" expression of femininity and sexuality was through reproduction and motherhood. Thus Cooke stated in 1943:

> The fundamental biologic factor in women is the reproductive urge of motherhood balanced by the fact that sexual pleasure is entirely secondary or even absent. . . . One of the commonest problems presented for solution by the gynecologist is the vast and fundamental difference between the sexes in regard to sexual appetite. Women with their almost *universal relative frigidity* are apt to react to the marital relationship in one of three ways. (A) They submit philosophically to their husbands. . . . (B) They submit rebelliously as a matter of duty. . . . (C) They rebel completely and through refusal try to force the husband to adapt himself to their own scale of sexual appetite [emphasis added]. [12]

Note that the unresponsiveness and resulting marital problems are exclusively the woman's fault, even though she is responding as she has been conditioned to respond, and even though to respond otherwise would be considered immoral or at least suspicious (nymphomania was a great concern). Second, any attempted adjustment on the part of the wife is treated as wrong and deleterious to the husband, while her own well-being is not a relevant variable.

Male sexuality, of course, is more important and of a much higher nature. Thus Cooke continues, "Biologically for the preservation of the race, the male is created to fertilize as many females as possible and hence is given an infinite appetite and capacity for intercourse."[13] Hence the basic chasm between the sexes: the male is in a constant quest to impregnate as many females as possible, for the good of the race, while the female paradoxically tries to avoid pregnancy in spite of her overpowering reproductive and maternal "instinct."

By the late forties, the stereotyped frigid female was an established fact among gynecologists. Treatment, instead of being directed toward the female, was designed to make intercourse more satisfying for the male and to remove any guilt or doubt that he may have had about his own competence and virility. From a 1952 text we learn:

> Unfortunate marital situations frequently arise because of the husband's resentment at the wife's sexual unresponsiveness. . . . It is good advice to recommend to the woman the advantage of *innocent simulation* of sex responsiveness, and as a matter of fact many women in their desire to please their husbands learned the advantage of such innocent deception [emphasis added].[14]

Novak's advice does not seem "innocent." It is another example of a way of keeping women down for men's benefit.

THE KINSEY ERA, 1953–1962

In 1953, Kinsey and Associates published *Sexual Behavior in the Human Female*. For the first time, the medical field had an authoritative and definitive (albeit based on a nonrandom sample) source of information on the female. For the most part, these texts used Kinsey's report selectively: findings which reinforced old stereotypes were repeated, while the revolutionary findings significant for women were ignored. For example, the textbooks often state that the male sets the sexual pace in marital coitus (of course, this is interpreted as "should set the pace"), but nowhere is it mentioned that women are multiorgasmic—a Kinsey finding which raises questions concerning the stronger male sex drive (and stronger usually implies superior).

Though Kinsey is not usually credited with the discovery, he debunked the myth of the vaginal orgasm. This finding should have put an end to the Freudian dictum that the clitoral orgasm, induced by masturbation or manipulation, is an immature response, while the vaginal orgasm, achievable only through intercourse, is the only mature sexual response. Kinsey stated that there are no nerve endings in the interior walls of the vagina; they are concentrated in the clitoris so that all sensations of orgasm must emanate from the clitoral region. He said, "The literature usually implies that the vagina itself should be the center of sensory stimulation but this as we have seen is a physical and physiologic impossibility for nearly all females."[15] Kinsey noted that some gynecologists, as early as 1942, were aware of the lack of nerves and end organs of touch in the vaginal surface. Quoting several doctors, he said, "This insensitivity of the vagina has been recognized by gynecologists who regularly probe and do surface operations in this area without using anesthesia. Under such conditions most patients show little if any awareness of pain."[16]

Gynecologists, however, tenaciously clung to the idea of the vaginal orgasm as the appropriate response. Since a great many women could not experience it, gynecologists continued to label their patients as sexually immature and therefore inferior to males sexually. For example, a 1956 text stated:

> Investigators of sexual behavior distinguish between clitoral and vaginal orgasms, the first playing a dominant role in childhood sexuality and in masturbation and the latter in the normal mature and sexually active woman. . . . The limitation of sexual satisfaction to one part of the external genitalia is apparently due to habit and aversion to normal cohabitation.[17]

Again we find the gynecologist defining normal sexuality for women in spite of concrete evidence to the contrary. Of course they knew that vaginal orgasms rarely occurred, but this was interpreted as the shortcoming of the individual female rather than as the gynecologist's reluctance to accept the research data. Indeed, as late as 1965 gynecology texts were reporting the vagina as the main erogenous zone.[18] In 1962:

> The transference of sensations from the clitoris to the vagina is completed only in part and frequently not at all. . . . If there has been much manual stimulation of the clitoris *it* may be reluctant to abandon control, or the vagina may be unwilling to accept the combined role of arbiter of sensation and vehicle for reproduction [emphasis added].[19]

The doctor seems to be involved in a form of projection in which the power struggle that he imagines between the clitoris and the vagina actually represents a parallel struggle between the sexes.

Another significant Kinsey finding had to do with the speed of sexual response in the female when manipulating the clitoris. The average was a few seconds under four minutes, with 45 percent of the sample achieving orgasm in under three minutes. Thus he concluded:

> There is widespread opinion that the female is slower than the male in her sexual responses, but the masturbatory data do not support that opinion. It is true that the average female responds more slowly than the average male in coitus but this seems to be due to the ineffectiveness of usual coital techniques.[20]

This might have suggested, especially to the medical scientist, that women should not be labeled frigid—a psychologically destructive word implying coldness and rigidity—but that the problem might lie in coital technique. However, the texts continued instead to make statements such as:

> Some women are truly frigid . . . psychic factors operate at the level of the cerebral cortex to inhibit the translation of sexual stimuli into a pleasurable response. Unless there is a true aversion to sex, the marital relations may proceed without *disturbing* either partner [emphasis added].[21]

Gynecology begins to look like medicine practiced on women for the benefit of men.

1962–PRESENT

In the early 1960s reports began to flow from the laboratories of Dr. William Masters and Ms. Virginia Johnson. Their findings

had more impact on the medical field than did Kinsey's, probably because their methods utilized scientific observation under controlled laboratory conditions. Masters and Johnson reinforced Kinsey's findings by adding a physiological analysis of sexual response, for example, in the detailed description of the four phases of the response cycle. While their findings are not generally directly quoted in gynecology texts, they have had an indirect influence, and by 1967 most texts had dropped the vaginal orgasm myth and began suggesting manipulation of the clitoris as part of foreplay.

With the favorite gynecologic misconceptions of vaginal orgasm and frigidity fairly well settled, textbook authors had to change their content somewhat. While the female orgasm can no longer be called inferior, or the lack of orgasm in intercourse be blamed on the female, she is still pictured as not as sexually potent as the male. In 1967 we read:

> In the woman sexual feelings are dormant as compared with those in the man and only develop gradually with experience. Extra-genital erotic sensations come easily but the desire for coitus and pleasure from it are acquired later.[22]

Explanations concerning the nature of the female core are also found frequently. Thus in 1967 we learn: "An important feature of sex desire in the man is the urge to dominate the woman and subjugate her to his will;[23] in the woman acquiescence to the masterful takes a high place."[24] Again, the female is defined as a nonaggressive, submissive, inferior being whose desire it is to be possessed by the powerful male. In 1971 we find this interpretation of the female personality:

> The traits that compose the core of the female personality are feminine narcissism, masochism, and passivity. The male traits of masculine narcissism, aggression, and activity lie at the other end of this spectrum.[25]

The author goes on to report that "every phase of a woman's life is influenced by narcissism."[26]

Finally, in cautioning women to watch their bowel habits, one gynecologist warns women against fitting the old definition that: "Woman is a constipated biped with a backache."[27]

The deleterious effect of such attitudes on the female patient can hardly be estimated. Certainly many women are aware of their powerless position in society and their expected passive, submissive behavior in the presence of a male.[28] But somehow you expect your doctor to be on your side or at least to try to see things from your perspective.

Thus we return to our original premise, that the basic underlying imagery of women has changed little in the past 125 years. The following two quotes are taken from two recent gynecology textbooks published in the United States. They contain the most current, yet the most ancient, male definition of female sexuality. In 1971, Dr. Thomas Green of Harvard wrote:

If the sexual inadequacy on the part of the wife stems from a fundamental immaturity and inability or failure to assume the normal adult female role in the marital relationship, he (the gynecologist) may be able to help by gradually imparting to her the nature of what her role should be—as Sturgis has described it so well, the fact that although the instinctive sexual drive of the male, who carries the primary responsibility for biologic survival of the race, is greater than hers, it is nevertheless of fundamental importance for the woman, his wife, particularly in a monogamous society, to make herself available for the fulfillment of this drive, and perfectly natural and normal that she do it willingly and derive satisfaction and pleasure from the union. Herein lies her power and purpose—to preserve the family unit as a happy, secure place for both man and wife and for the rearing of their children. Only by understanding and assuming this role can a woman throw off childhood inhibitions and taboos and attain the feminine maturity essential to a happy, successful marital adjustment.[29]

In *Novak's Textbook of Gynecology* (1970), we are told:

The frequency of intercourse depends entirely upon the male sex drive. . . . The bride should be advised to allow her husband's sex drive to set their pace and she should attempt to gear hers satisfactorily to his. If she finds after several months or years that this is not possible, she is advised to consult her Physician as soon as she realizes there is a real problem. In assuming this role of "follow the leader," however, she is cautioned not to make her sexual relations completely passive. Certain overt advances are attractive and provocative and active participation in the sex act is necessary for full

fruition. She may be reminded that it is unsatisfactory to take a tone-deaf individual to a concert.[30]

CONCLUSIONS: AFTER READING GYNECOLOGY TEXTS

> The perspective is for men
> In the field of G Y N.
> You will find your pleasure tiny
> If you read your OB Gyne.
> And to learn you're full of sin
> Read the work of OB Gyn.
> So just recall, tho tears it brings
> That man's the measure of all things.
>
> Pauline Bart

NOTES

1. For a detailed discussion of medical training in obstetrics and gynecology, see Diana Scully, "Obstetrics and Gynecology: Social Processes in Skill Acquisition and Implications for Patient Care" (Ph.D. diss., University of Illinois at Chicago Circle, 1977).
2. Dr. Lésère Colombat, *Colombat on the Diseases of Females: A Treatise on the Diseases and Special Hygiene of Females,** with translation and additions by Charles D. Meigs (Philadelphia: Lea and Blanchard, 1845), p. 542.
3. C. D. Meigs, "Females and Their Diseases: A Series of Letters to His Classes" (1848), cited in Milton Abramson, "Preparation for Marriage and Parenthood," in *Psychosomatic Obstetrics, Gynecology and Endocrinology,** ed. William S. Kroger (Springfield, Ill.: C. Thomas, 1962).
4. With few exceptions such as: E. Stewart Taylor, *Essentials of Gynecology** (Philadelphia: Lea Febiger, 1962); and David Danforth, *Textbook of Obstetrics and Gynecology** (New York: Hoeber, 1971).
5. Taylor, *Essentials of Gynecology*.
6. Ibid.
7. For a general article on sexism in the social sciences, see Pauline Bart, "Sexism and Social Science: From the Gilded Cage to the Iron

---

* Indicates one of the twenty-eight gynecology textbooks used in this study.

Cage, or, the Perils of Pauline," *Journal of Marriage and the Family* 33 (1971): 734–45. For sociology, see Jessie Bernard, "Letter to the American Sociologist," *American Sociologist* 5 (1970): 374–75; and Alice Rossi, "Women in the 70's; Problems and Possibilities," paper presented at Barnard College (1970). For history, see Ruth Rosen, "Sexism in History, or, Writing Women's History Is a Tricky Business," *Journal of Marriage and the Family* 33 (1971): 541–44. For marriage and the family books, see Carol Ehrlich, "The Male Sociologist's Burden: The Place of Women in Marriage and Family Texts," *Journal of Marriage and the Family* 33 (1971): 421–30. For marriage manuals, see Penelope J. Shankweiler and Michael Gordon, "Different Equals Less: Female Sexuality in Recent Marriage Manuals," *Journal of Marriage and the Family* 33 (1971): 459–66. For preschool and elementary school texts, see Lenore J. Weitzman, Deborah Eifler, Elizabeth Hakeda, and Catherine Ross, "Sex Role Socialization in Children's Picture Books," paper presented to the American Sociological Association, September 1971; and see also Marjorie B. U'Ren, "The Image of Woman in Textbooks," in *Woman in Sexist Society*, ed. Vivian Gornick and Barbara K. Moran (New York: Basic Books, 1971).

8. Two surveys made during the sixties by the American College of Obstetrics and Gynecology report that "93% of general practitioners, internists, obstetricians, and gynecologists are treating marital and sexual problems of patients. Only 15% felt that either medical school or residency had adequately prepared them to do this. 90% to 95% felt that more training was needed to prepare today's physician to cope with those marital problems which contribute to the current social dilemma and result in psychosomatic and organic disease." See Ethel M. Nash, "Divorce: Marriage Counseling," in *The Social Responsibility of Obstetrics and Gynecology*,* ed. Allen C. Barnes (Baltimore: The Johns Hopkins Press, 1965), pp. 117–18. See also Edmund R. Novak, Georgeanna Seegar Jones, and Howard W. Jones, *Novak's Textbook of Gynecology** (Baltimore: The Williams and Wilkens Co., 1970), and Thomas H. Green, *Gynecology: Essentials of Clinical Practice** (Boston: Little, Brown, 1971).

9. We do not mean to deny the importance of meaningful scientific advances within the field of gynecology and obstetrics. The maternal death rate *has* declined sharply. Yet the obstetricians did not heed Semmelweiss' advice to wash their hands to prevent puerperal fever, and in the forties and fifties the number of unnecessary hys-

terectomies was a scandal. One physician (not a gynecologist) said to Bart, "All women over forty-five should have hysterectomies prophylactically" (presumably to prevent cancer). Would he have suggested that all males over fifty have their prostates removed prophylactically?

10. Emil Novak and Edmund R. Novak, *Textbook of Gynecology** (Baltimore: The Williams and Wilkens Co., 1952), p. 572.
11. C. Russell Scott, *The World of a Gynecologist** (London: Oliver and Boyd, 1968), p. 25.
12. Willard R. Cooke, *Essentials of Gynecology** (Philadelphia: J. B. Lippincott Co., 1943), pp. 59–60.
13. Ibid., p. 60.
14. Novak and Novak, *Textbook of Gynecology*, p. 572.
15. Alfred C. Kinsey et al., *Sexual Behavior in the Human Female* (New York: Simon & Schuster, 1953), p. 582.
16. Ibid., p. 580.
17. I. C. Rubin and Josef Novak, *Integrated Gynecology: Principles and Practice,** vol. III (New York: McGraw-Hill, 1956), p. 77.
18. J. P. Greenhill, *Office Gynecology** (Chicago: Yearbook Medical Publishers, Inc., 1965), p. 496.
19. Langdon Parsons and Sheldon C. Sommers, *Gynecology** (Philadelphia: W. B. Saunders Co., 1962), pp. 501–2.
20. Kinsey et al., *Sexual Behavior in the Human Female*, p. 164.
21. Parsons and Sommers, *Gynecology*, p. 494.
22. Thomas Jeffcoate, *Principles of Gynecology** (London: Butterworth, 1967), p. 726.
23. It is interesting to note that radical feminists take a similar position: sex is a male power trip. See Susan Griffin, "Rape: The All American Crime," *Ramparts Magazine* (September 1971).
24. Jeffcoate, *Principles of Gynecology*, p. 726.
25. James Robert Willson, *Obstetrics and Gynecology** (St. Louis: Mosby, 1971), p. 43.
26. Ibid.
27. Greenhill, *Office Gynecology*, p. 194.
28. S. L. Bem and D. J. Bem, "Case Study of a Nonconscious Ideology: Training the Woman to Know Her Place," in D. J. Bem, *Belief, Attitudes and Human Affairs* (Belmont, California: Brooks/Cole, 1970).
29. Green, *Gynecology: Essentials of Clinical Practice*, p. 436.
30. Novak, Jones, and Jones, *Novak's Textbook of Gynecology*, pp. 662–63.

ADDITIONAL REFERENCES

Pauline Bart and Linda Frankel, *The Student Sociologist's Handbook* (Cambridge, Mass.: Schenkman Publishers, 1971).

Samuel J. Behrman and John R. C. Gosling, *Fundamentals of Gynecology** (New York: Oxford University Press, 1959).

Ralph C. Benson, *Handbook of Obstetrics and Gynecology** (Los Altos, California: Lange Medical Publishers, 1971).

Ruth Brecher and Edward Brecher, eds., *An Analysis of Human Sexual Response* (New York: The New American Library, 1966).

John I. Brewer and Edwin J. DeCosta, *Textbook of Gynecology** (Baltimore: The Williams and Wilkens Co., 1967).

Robert James Crossen, *Diseases of Women** (St. Louis: C. V. Mosby Co., 1953).

A. H. Curtis, *A Textbook of Gynecology** (Philadelphia: W. B. Saunders, 1946).

Henry Carl Davis, "Premarital Education, Examination, and Advice," in *Gynecology and Obstetrics*,* vol. III ed. Carl Henry Davis, (Hagerstown, Md.: W. F. Prior Co., 1964).

William Filler, "Normal and Abnormal Sex Problems and Practices," in *Gynecology: Diseases and Minor Surgery*,* ed. Robert J. Lowrie (Springfield, Ill.: C. Thomas, 1952).

Cornelia Butler Flora, "The Passive Female: Her Comparative Image by Class and Culture in Women's Magazine Fiction," *Journal of Marriage and the Family* 33 (1971): 435–44.

John William Huffman, *Gynecology and Obstetrics** (Philadelphia: W. B. Saunders, 1962).

R. W. Kistner, *Gynecology** (Chicago: Yearbook Medical Publishers, Inc., 1964).

R. D. Laing, *Self and Others* (Middlesex, England: Penguin Books, 1961).

Alfred C. Ludwig, B. J. Murowski, and Somers H. Sturgis, *Psychosomatic Aspects of Gynecology** (Cambridge, Mass.: Harvard University Press, 1969).

J. V. Meigs and S. H. Sturgis, *Progress in Gynecology** (New York: Grune and Stratton, 1963).

Mary De Witt Pettit, *Gynecologic Diagnosis and Treatment** (New York: McGraw-Hill, 1962).

G. D. Pinker and D. W. T. Roberts, *A Short Textbook of Obstetrics and Gynecology** (Philadelphia: Lippincott, 1967).

Walter Reich and M. Wechtow, *Practical Gynecology** (Philadelphia: Lippincott, 1957).

Clara Thompson, "Some Effects of the Derogatory Attitude Toward Female Sexuality," in *Psychoanalysis and Female Sexuality*, ed. Hendrik M. Ruitenbeek (New Haven, Conn.: College and University Press, 1966).

Time Magazine, "Situation Report," March 20, 1972, p. 89.

L. R. Wharton, *Gynecology** (Philadelphia: W. B. Saunders, 1943).

PART 3

MEDICINE AND
IMPERIALISM: OF YOU
THE STORY IS TOLD

FRANTZ FANON
MEDICINE AND COLONIALISM

THE ALGERIAN EXAMPLE

Introduced into Algeria at the same time as racialism and humiliation, Western medical science, being part of the oppressive system, has always provoked in the native an ambivalent attitude. This ambivalence is in fact to be found in connection with all of the occupier's modes of presence. With medicine we come to one of the most tragic features of the colonial situation.

In all objectivity and in all humanity, it is a good thing that a technically advanced country benefits from its knowledge and the discoveries of its scientists. When the discipline considered concerns man's health, when its very principle is to ease pain, it is clear that no negative reaction can be justified. But the colonial situation is precisely such that it drives the colonized to appraise all the colonizer's contributions in a pejorative and absolute way. The colonized perceives the doctor, the engineer, the schoolteacher, the policeman, the rural constable, through the haze of an almost organic confusion. The compulsory visit by the doctor to the *douar* is preceded by the assembling of the population through the agency of the police authorities. The doctor who arrives in this atmosphere of general constraint is never a native doctor but always a doctor belonging to the dominant society and very often to the army.

The statistics on sanitary improvements are not interpreted by the native as progress in the fight against illness, in general, but as fresh proof of the extension of the occupier's hold on the country. When the French authorities show visitors through the Tizi-Ouzou sanatorium or the operating units of the Mustapha hospital

in Algiers, this has for the native just one meaning: "This is what we have done for the people of this country; this country owes us everything; were it not for us, there would be no country." There is a real mental reservation on the part of the native; it is difficult for him to be objective, to separate the wheat from the chaff.

There are of course exceptions. In certain periods of calm, in certain free confrontations, the colonized individual frankly recognizes what is positive in the dominator's action. But this good faith is immediately taken advantage of by the occupier and transformed into a justification of the occupation. When the native, after a major effort in the direction of truth, because he assumes that his defenses have been surmounted, says, "That is good. I tell you so because I think so," the colonizer perverts his meaning and translates, "Don't leave, for what would we do without you?"

Thus, on the level of the whole colonized society, we always discover this reluctance to qualify opposition to the colonialist, for it so happens that every qualification is perceived by the occupier as an invitation to perpetuate the oppression, as a confession of congenital impotence. The colonized people as a whole, when faced with certain happenings, will react in a harsh, undifferentiated, categorical way before the dominant group's activity. It is not unusual to hear such extreme observations as this: "Nobody asked you for anything; who invited you to come? Take your hospitals and your port facilities and go home."

The fact is that the colonization, having been built on military conquest and the police system, sought a justification for its existence and the legitimization of its persistence in its works.

Reduced, in the name of truth and reason, to saying "yes" to certain innovations of the occupier, the colonized perceived that he thus became the prisoner of the entire system, and that the French medical service in Algeria could not be separated from French colonialism in Algeria. Then, as he could not cut himself off from his people, who aspired to a national existence on their own soil, he rejected doctors, schoolteachers, engineers, parachutists, all in one lump.

In a noncolonial society, the attitude of a sick man in the presence of a medical practitioner is one of confidence. The patient

trusts the doctor; he puts himself in his hands. He yields his body to him. He accepts the fact that pain may be awakened or exacerbated by the physician, for the patient realizes that the intensifying of suffering in the course of examination may pave the way to peace in his body.

At no time, in a noncolonial society, does the patient mistrust his doctor. On the level of technique, of knowledge, it is clear that a certain doubt can filter into the patient's mind, but this may be due to a hesitation on the part of the doctor which modifies the original confidence. This can happen anywhere. But it is obvious that certain circumstances can appreciably change the doctor-patient relationship. The German prisoner who was to be operated on by a French surgeon would very often, just before being given the anaesthetic, beseech the doctor not to kill him. Under the same circumstances, the surgeon might be more than ordinarily anxious to perform the operation successfully because of the other prisoners, because he realized the interpretation that might be given the event if a patient died on the operating table. The French prisoners in the German camps showed a similar concern when they asked the doctors working in the camp infirmary to assist in the operations performed by German surgeons. Literature and the motion pictures have made much of such situations, and after every war the problems they involve are commercially exploited.

In colonial territory such situations are to be found in even greater number. The sudden deaths of Algerians in hospitals, a common occurrence in any establishment caring for the sick and the injured, are interpreted as the effects of a murderous and deliberate decision, as the result of criminal maneuvers on the part of the European doctor. The Algerian's refusal to be hospitalized is always more or less related to that lingering doubt as to the colonial doctor's essential humanity. It needs to be said, too, although it is not the rule, that in certain hospital services experimentation on living patients is practiced to an extent that cannot be considered negligible.[1]

For dozens of years, despite the doctor's exhortations, the Algerian shied away from hospitalization. Even though the specialist might insist that any hesitation would seriously en-

danger the patient's life, the patient would hang back and refuse to be taken to the hospital. It would always be at the last moment, when hardly any hope remained, that consent was given. Even then, the man who made the decision would make it in opposition to the group; and as the case would be a desperate one, as the decision had been too long delayed, the patient would usually die.

Such experiences would strengthen the group in its original belief in the occupier's fundamentally evil character, even though he was a doctor. And the Algerian who, after considerable effort, had succeeded in overcoming the traditional prejudice to an appreciable extent, who had forced the decision to hospitalize the patient, would suddenly feel infinitely guilty. Inwardly he would promise not to repeat his mistake. The values of the group, momentarily abandoned, would reassert themselves, in an exacerbated and exclusive way.

It would be a serious mistake, and it would in any case make such an attitude incomprehensible, to compare such behavior with that already described as characterizing the poor rural populations of European countries. The colonized who resisted hospitalization did not do so on the basis of the fear of cities, the fear of distance, of no longer being protected by the family, the fear that people would say that the patient had been sent to the hospital to die, that the family had rid itself of a burden. The colonized not only refused to send the patient to the hospital, but he refused to send him to the hospital of the whites, of strangers, of the conqueror.

It is necessary to analyze, patiently and lucidly, each one of the reactions of the colonized, and every time we do not understand, we must tell ourselves that we are at the heart of the drama—that of the impossibility of finding a meeting ground in any colonial situation. For some time it was maintained that the native's reluctance to entrust himself to a European doctor was due to his attachment to his traditional medical techniques or to his dependence on the sorcerers or healers of his group. Such psychological reactions do obviously exist, and they were to be observed, not too many years ago, not only among the masses of generally advanced countries, but also among doctors them-

selves. Leriche has reported to us the hesitancies or the refusals of certain doctors to adopt the thermometer because they were accustomed to estimating the temperature by taking the pulse. Examples of this kind could be indefinitely multiplied. It is hardly abnormal, therefore, for individuals accustomed to practicing certain customs in the treatment of a given ailment, to adopting certain procedures when confronted with the disorder that illness constitutes, to refuse to abandon these customs and procedures because others are imposed on them, in other words because the new technique takes over completely and does not tolerate the persistence of any shred of tradition.

Here again we hear the same refrain: "If I abandon what I am in the habit of doing when my wife coughs and I authorize the European doctor to give her injections; if I find myself literally insulted and told I am a savage [this happens], because I have made scratches on the forehead of my son who has been complaining of a headache for three days; if I tell this insulter he is right and I admit that I was wrong to make those scratches which custom has taught me to do—if I do all these things I am acting, from a strictly rational point of view, in a positive way. For, as a matter of fact, my son has meningitis and it really has to be treated as a meningitis ought to be treated. But the colonial constellation is such that what should be the brotherly and tender insistence of one who wants only to help me is interpreted as a manifestation of the conqueror's arrogance and desire to humiliate."

It is not possible for the colonized society and the colonizing society to agree to pay tribute, at the same time and in the same place, to a single value. If, against all probability, the colonized society expresses its agreement on any point with the colonizing society, there will at once begin to be talk about successful integration. It is now necessary to enter into the tragic labyrinth of the general reactions of Algerian society with respect to the problem of the fight against illness, conceived of as an aspect of the French presence. We shall then see in the course of the fight for liberation the crystallization of the new attitude adopted by the Algerian people in respect to medical techniques.

THE VISIT TO THE DOCTOR

The colonized person who goes to see the doctor is always diffident. He answers in monosyllables, gives little in the way of explanation, and soon arouses the doctor's impatience. This attitude is not to be confused with the kind of inhibiting fear that patients usually feel in the doctor's presence. We often hear it said that a certain doctor has a good bedside manner, that he puts his patients at ease. But it so happens that in the colonial situation the personal approach, the ability to be oneself, of establishing and maintaining a "contact," are not observable. The colonial situation standardizes relations, for it dichotomizes the colonial society in a marked way.

The doctor rather quickly gave up the hope of obtaining information from the colonized patient and fell back on the clinical examination, thinking that the body would be more eloquent. But the body proved to be equally rigid. The muscles were contracted. There was no relaxing. Here was the entire man, here was the colonized, facing both a technician and a colonizer.[2] One must, of course, lend an ear to the observations made by the European doctors who examined the patients. But one must also hear those of the patients themselves when they left the hospital. Whereas the *doctors* say: "The pain in their case is protopathic, poorly differentiated, diffuse as in an animal, it is a general malaise rather than a localized pain"; the *patients* say: "They asked me what was wrong with me, as if I were the doctor; they think they're smart and they aren't even able to tell where I feel pain, and the minute you come in they ask you what is wrong with you . . ."

The doctors say: "Those people are rough and unmannerly." The patients say: "I don't trust them." Whereas the doctors claim that the colonized patient doesn't know what he wants, whether to stay sick or be cured, the native keeps saying, "I know how to get into their hospital, but I don't know how I'll get out—*if* I get out." Fairly soon the doctor, and even the nurse, worked out a rule of action: with these people you couldn't practice medicine, you had to be a veterinarian.[3] But finally, by sheer persistence, the doctor would more or less get an idea of what the disease was

and prescribe a treatment, which would sometimes not be followed. Sociologists would thereupon venture an explanation and classify all these actions under the heading of fatalism.

The analysis of this pattern of behavior within the colonial framework enables us, on the contrary, to come to other conclusions.

When the colonized escapes the doctor, and the integrity of his body is preserved, he considers himself the victor by a handsome margin. For the native the visit is always an ordeal. When the advantage assumed by the colonizer is limited to swallowing pills or potions, the colonized has the impression of having won a victory over the enemy. The end of the visit puts an end to the confrontation. The medicines, the advice, are but the sequels of the ordeal. As for fatalism, a father's apparent refusal, for example, to admit that he owes his son's life to the colonizer's operation, must be studied in two lights. There is, first of all, the fact that the colonized person, who in this respect is like the men in underdeveloped countries or the disinherited in all parts of the world, perceives life not as a flowering or a development of an essential productiveness, but as a permanent struggle against an omnipresent death. This ever-menacing death is experienced as endemic famine, unemployment, a high death rate, an inferiority complex, and the absence of any hope for the future.

All this gnawing at the existence of the colonized tends to make of life something resembling an incomplete death. Acts of refusal or rejection of medical treatment are not a refusal of life, but a greater passivity before that close and contagious death. Seen from another angle, this absence of enlightened behavior reveals the colonized native's mistrust of the colonizing technician. The technician's words are always understood in a pejorative way. The truth objectively expressed is constantly vitiated by the lie of the colonial situation.

MEDICAL SUPERVISION, TREATMENT, AND THE "DOUBLE-POWER"

A poor subject in the doctor's office, the colonized Algerian proves to be an equally unsatisfactory patient. The colonizing

doctor finds that his patient cannot be depended upon to take his medicine regularly, that he takes the wrong doses, fails to appreciate the importance of periodic visits, and takes a paradoxical, frivolous attitude toward the prescribed diet. These are only the most striking and the most common peculiarities that he notes. Hence the general impression that the patient plays hide-and-seek with his doctor. The doctor has no hold on the patient. He finds that in spite of promises and pledges, an attitude of flight, of disengagement persists. All the efforts exerted by the doctor, by his team of nurses, to modify this state of things encounter, not a systematic opposition, but a "vanishing" on the part of the patient.

The first thing that happens is that the patient does not return. This in spite of the fact that it has been clearly explained to him that his ailment, in order to be cured, requires that he be examined several times at given intervals. This is clearly written out in the prescription, it has been explained to him and reexplained, and he has been given a definite appointment with the doctor for a fixed date. But the doctor waits for him in vain. The patient does not arrive. When he does come back, there is the rather shocking discovery that the malady has become very much aggravated. The patient, in fact, comes back five to six months or sometimes a year later. Worse still, he has failed to take the prescribed medicine. An interview with the patient reveals that the medicine was taken only once, or, as often happens, that the amount prescribed for one month was absorbed in a single dose. It may be worthwhile to dwell on this type of case, for the explanations of it that have been given appear to us quite unsatisfactory.

The sociological theory is that the "native" entertains the firm hope of being cured once and for all. The native, in fact, sees the ailment not as progressing little by little but as assaulting the individual in a single swoop, so that the effectiveness of a remedy would not depend so much on its consistent, periodic, and progressive repetition but on its total impact, its immediate effect; this accounts for the natives' preference for injections. According to this theory, the doctor would always have to heal at a single sitting. Pilgrimages to a sanctuary, the making of amulets or marks written on a piece of paper—these are therapies that are

applied immediately with the maximum effectiveness. Just as neglecting a ritual duty or transgressing a given taboo causes the disease to break out, so performing certain actions or following the medicine man's or the sorcerer's prescriptions are capable of expelling the disease and restoring the equilibrium between the different forces that govern the life of the group.

This explanation surely contains an element of truth. But it seems to us that to interpret a phenomenon arising out of the colonial situation in terms of patterns of conduct existing before the foreign conquest, even if this phenomenon is analogous to certain traditional patterns, is nevertheless in certain respects false. Colonial domination, as we have seen, gives rise to and continues to dictate a whole complex of resentful behavior and of refusal on the part of the colonized. The colonized exerts a considerable effort to keep away from the colonial world, not to expose himself to any action of the conqueror. In everyday life, however, the colonized and the colonizers are constantly establishing bonds of economic, technical, and administrative dependence. Colonialism obviously throws all the elements of native society into confusion. The dominant group arrives with its values and imposes them with such violence that the very life of the colonized can manifest itself only defensively, in a more or less clandestine way. Under these conditions, colonial domination distorts the very relations that the colonized maintains with his own culture. In a great number of cases, the practice of tradition is a disturbed practice, the colonized being unable to reject completely modern discoveries and the arsenal of weapons against diseases possessed by the hospitals, the ambulances, the nurses. But the colonized who accepts the intervention of medical technique, if he does not go to the hospital, will be subjected to considerable pressure on the part of his group. The traditional methods of treatment are applied in addition to the modern medical technique. "Two remedies are better than one." It must be remembered that the colonized who accepts penicillin or digitalin at the same time insists on following the treatment prescribed by the healer of his village or his district.

The colonized obscurely realizes that penicillin is more effective, but for political, psychological, social reasons, he must at the same time give traditional medicine its due. (The healer fulfills a

function and therefore needs to earn a living.) Psychologically, the colonized has difficulty, even here in the presence of illness, in rejecting the habits of his group and the reactions of his culture. Accepting the medicine, even once, is admitting, to a limited extent perhaps but nonetheless ambiguously, the validity of the Western technique. It is demonstrating one's confidence in the foreigner's medical science. Swallowing the whole dose in one gulp is literally getting even with it.

To adopt gradually an almost obsessional respect for the colonizer's prescription often proves difficult. The other power, in fact, intervenes and breaks the unifying circle of the Western therapy. Every pill absorbed or every injection taken invites the application of a preparation or the visit to a saint. Sometimes the patient gives evidence of the fear of being the battleground for different and opposed forces. This fear gives rise to important stresses and the whole picture of the illness is thereby modified. Once again, the colonial world reveals itself to be complex and extremely diverse in structure. There is always an opposition of exclusive worlds, a contradictory interaction of different techniques, a vehement confrontation of values.

THE COLONIZED AND THE NATIVE DOCTOR

The colonial situation does not only vitiate the relations between doctor and patient. We have shown that the doctor always appears as a link in the colonialist network, as a spokesman for the occupying power. We shall see that this ambivalence of the patient before medical technique is to be found even when the doctor belongs to the dominated people. There is a manifest ambivalence of the colonized group with respect to any member who acquires a technique or the manners of the conqueror. For the group, in fact, the native technician is living proof that any one of its members is capable of being an engineer, a lawyer or a doctor. But there is at the same time, in the background, the awareness of a sudden divergence between the homogeneous group, enclosed within itself, and this native technician who has escaped beyond the specific psychological or emotional categories of the people. The native doctor is a Europeanized, Westernized doctor, and in certain circumstances he is consid-

ered as no longer being a part of the dominated society. He is tacitly rejected into the camp of the oppressors, into the opposing camp. It is not by accident that in certain colonies the educated native is referred to as "having acquired the habits of a master."

For many of the colonized, the native doctor is compared to the native police, to the *caïd*, to the notable. The colonized is both proud of the success of his *race* and at the same time looks upon this technician with disapproval. The native doctor's behavior with respect to the traditional medicine of his country is for a long time characterized by a considerable aggressiveness.

The native doctor feels himself psychologically compelled to demonstrate firmly his new admission to a rational universe. This accounts for the abrupt way in which he rejects the magic practices of his people. Given the ambivalence of the colonized with respect to the native doctor and the ambivalence of the native doctor before certain features of his culture, the encounter of doctor and patient inevitably proves difficult. The colonized patient is the first to set the tone. Once the superiority of Western technique over traditional methods of treatment is recognized, it is thought preferable to turn to the colonizers who are, after all, "the true possessors of the technique." As far as practice goes, it is common to see European doctors receiving both Algerian and European patients, whereas Algerian doctors generally receive only Algerians. Some exceptions could of course be mentioned; but on the whole, this description is valid for Algeria. The native doctor, because of the operation of the complex psychological laws that govern colonial society, frequently finds himself in a difficult position.

We are dealing here with the drama of the colonized intellectuals *before* the fight for liberation. We shall soon see what important modifications have been introduced into Algeria by the national war of liberation.

THE EUROPEAN DOCTOR DURING THE STRUGGLE FOR LIBERATION

Generally speaking, the colonizing doctor adopts the attitude of his group toward the struggle of the Algerian people. Behind "the doctor who heals the wounds of humanity" appears the man,

a member of a dominant society and enjoying in Algeria the benefit of an incomparably higher standard of living than that of his metropolitan colleague.[4]

Moreover, in centers of colonization the doctor is nearly always a landowner as well. It is exceptional to see in Algeria, a colony which attracts settlers, a doctor who does not take up farming, who does not become attached to the soil. Whether the land has come to him from his family, or he has bought it himself, the doctor is a settler. The European population in Algeria has not yet clearly marked out for itself the different sectors of economic life. Colonial society is a mobile society, poorly structured, and the European, even when he is a technician, always assumes a certain degree of polyvalence. In the heart of every European in the colonies there slumbers a man of energy, a pioneer, an adventurer. Not even the civil servant transferred for two years to a colonial territory fails to feel himself psychologically changed in certain respects.

The European individual in Algeria does not take his place in a structured and relatively stable society. The colonial society is in perpetual movement. Every settler invents a new society, sets up or sketches new structures. The differences between craftsmen, civil servants, workers, and professionals are poorly defined. Every doctor has his vineyards and the lawyer busies himself with his rice fields as passionately as any settler. The doctor is not socially defined by the exercise of his profession alone. He is likewise the owner of mills, wine cellars, or orange groves, and he coyly speaks of his medicine as simply a supplementary source of income. Not exclusively dependent on his practice, deriving a sometimes enormous income from his properties, the doctor has a certain conception of professional morality and of medical practice. The colonialist arrogance, the contempt for the client, the hateful brutality toward the indigent are more or less contained in the formula, "I don't have to sit around waiting for clients to make a living." The doctor in Besançon, in Liège, or in Basel has left the land and has taken his place in the economic sector defined by his profession. Perpetually in contact with suffering humanity, the world of the sick and the disabled, the doctor has a set of values. Thus he will usually be found to belong

to one of the democratic parties, and his ideas are likely to be anticolonialist. In the colonies, the doctor is an integral part of colonization, of domination, of exploitation. In Algeria we must not be surprised to find that doctors and professors of medicine are leaders of colonialist movements.

The Algerian doctor is economically interested in the maintenance of colonial oppression. This is not a question of values or of principles, but of the incomparably high standard of living that the colonial situation provides him. This explains the fact that very often he assumes the role of militia chief or organizer of "counterterrorist" raids. In the colonies, in normal times—that is, in the absence of the war of liberation—there is something of the cowboy and the pioneer even in the intellectual. In a period of crisis the cowboy pulls out his revolver and his instruments of torture.

In this frightful war that is bathing Algeria in blood, an effort is required to understand certain facts, objectively distressing in a normal situation. The murder of certain doctors in Algeria has never been clearly understood by world opinion. In the cruelest wars, it is traditional for the medical corps to be left unscathed. For example, in 1944, while freeing a village in the region of Belfort, we left a guard at the entrance to a school where German surgeons were operating on the wounded. The Algerian political men are quite aware of the existence of laws of war. They know the complexity of the problem and the dramatic situation of the European population. How is one to explain those cases, the decisions made to take the life of a doctor?

It is almost always because the doctor himself, by his behavior, has decided to exclude himself from the protective circle that the principles and the values of the medical profession have woven around him. The doctor who is killed in Algeria, in isolated cases, is always a war criminal. In a colonial situation there are special realities. In a given region, the doctor sometimes reveals himself as the most sanguinary of colonizers. His identity as a doctor no longer matters. Just as he was a doctor in addition to being a property owner, so he becomes the torturer who happens to be a doctor. The dominant authority, for that matter, has organized the overall behavior of the doctor as it relates to the struggle for

liberation. Thus, any doctor treating an Algerian whose wound appears suspicious must, on penalty of legal action, take down the name of the patient, his address, the names of those accompanying him, their addresses, and communicate the information to the authorities.[5]

As for the pharmacists, they were to be given orders not to deliver without a medical prescription such drugs as penicillin, streptomycin, antibiotics in general, alcohol, absorbent cotton, anti-tetanus serum. Moreover, they were strongly urged to note down the identity and the address of the patient.

As soon as they were known to the people, these measures confirmed their certainty that the colonizers were in complete agreement to fight against them. Convinced that the European doctors and pharmacists would comply with this decision, the French authorities posted police officers in civilian clothes or informers in the vicinity of the pharmacies run by Algerians. The supplying of medicines in certain areas became a difficult and painful problem. Alcohol, sulpha drugs, syringes were refused. In 1955, the French military command in its estimates of Algerian losses nearly always included a certain number of hypothetically wounded who, "for lack of treatment are assumed dead."

The colonizing doctor, meanwhile, emphasized his membership in the dominating society by certain attitudes. When judicial inquiries into the cases of Algerians who had not died in the course of police questioning began, it would happen that the defense would ask for a medico-legal examination. This demand would sometimes be met. The European doctor assigned to examine the patient always concluded that there was no evidence to suggest that the accused had been tortured. A few times, early in 1955, Algerians were appointed as experts. But precise instructions prohibiting this were soon issued. Likewise, if it happened that a European doctor noted "the existence of elements that might suggest the hypothesis that acts described by the accused produced his wounds," another expert opinion was immediately found to contradict him. Obviously, such a doctor was never called in again. Not infrequently the European doctor in Algeria would deliver to the legal authority a certificate of natural death for an Algerian who had succumbed to torture or who, more

simply, had been coldly executed. Similarly, it invariably happened that when the demand of the defense for an autopsy was granted, the results would be negative.

On the strictly technical level, the European doctor actively collaborates with the colonial forces in their most frightful and most degrading practices. We should like to mention here some of the practices engaged in by the European medical corps in Algeria, which shed light on certain "murders" of doctors.

First of all, the "truth serum." The principle of this drug is well known: a chemical substance having hypnotic properties is injected into a vein, which, when the operation is carried out slowly, produces a certain loss of control, a blunting of consciousness. As a therapeutic measure used in medicine it is obviously a very dangerous technique, which may cause a serious impairment of the personality. Many psychiatrists, considering the dangers greater than the possible improvements, have long ago abandoned this technique for examining spheres of the unconscious.

All the academies of medicine of all the countries in the world have formally condemned the use of this practice for legal ends and the doctor who violates these solemn proscriptions is obviously contemptuous of the fundamental principles of medicine. The doctor who fights side by side with his people, as a doctor, must respect the international charter of his profession. A criminal doctor, in all countries in the world, is sentenced to death. The example of the doctors in the human experimentation camps of the Nazis is particularly edifying.

The European doctors in Algeria use the "truth serum" with staggering frequency. We may recall here the experience of Henri Alleg, as related in *The Question*.[6]

We have had occasion to treat men and women who had been subjected to this torture for days. We shall study elsewhere the grave consequences of these practices, but we can point out here that the most important consequence has appeared to us to be a certain inability to distinguish the true from the false, and an almost obsessive fear of saying what should remain hidden. We must always remember that there is hardly an Algerian who is not a party to at least one secret of the revolution. Months after this

torture, the former prisoner hesitates to say his name, the town where he was born. Every question is first experienced as a repetition of the torturer-tortured relationship.

Other doctors, attached to the various torture centers, intervene after every session in order to put the tortured back into condition for new sessions. Under the circumstances, the important thing is for the prisoner not to give the slip to the team in charge of the questioning: in other words, to remain alive. Everything—heart stimulants, massive doses of vitamins—is used before, during, and after the sessions to keep the Algerian hovering between life and death. Ten times the doctor intervenes, ten times he gives the prisoner back to the pack of torturers.

In the European medical corps in Algeria, and especially in the military health corps, such things are common. Professional morality, medical ethics, self-respect, and respect for others have given way to the most uncivilized, the most degrading, the most perverse kinds of behavior. Finally, attention must be called to the habit formed by certain psychiatrists of flying to the aid of the police. There are, for instance, psychiatrists in Algiers, known to numerous prisoners, who have given electric shock treatments to the accused and have questioned them during the waking phase, which is characterized by a certain confusion, a relaxation of resistance, a disappearance of the person's defenses. When by chance these men are liberated because the doctor, despite this barbarous treatment, was able to obtain no information, what is brought to us is a personality in shreds. The work of rehabilitating the man is then extremely difficult. This is only one of the numerous crimes of which French colonialism in Algeria has made itself guilty.[7]

THE ALGERIAN PEOPLE, MEDICAL TECHNIQUE,
AND THE WAR OF LIBERATION

We have had occasion many times to point out the appearance of radically new types of behavior in various aspects of the private and public life of the Algerian. The shock that broke the chains of colonialism has moderated exclusive attitudes, reduced extreme positions, made certain arbitrary views obsolete. Medical science

and concern for one's health have always been proposed or imposed by the occupying power. In the colonial situation, however, it is impossible to create the physical and psychological conditions for the learning of hygiene or for the assimilation of concepts concerning epidemic diseases. In the colonial situation, going to see the doctor, the administrator, the constable, or the mayor are identical moves. The sense of alienation from colonial society and the mistrust of the representatives of its authority are always accompanied by an almost mechanical sense of detachment and mistrust of even the things that are most positive and most profitable to the population.

We have noted that in the very first months of the struggle, the French authorities decided to put an embargo on antibiotics, ether, alcohol, anti-tetanus vaccine. The Algerian who wished to obtain any of these medications was required to give the pharmacist detailed information as to his identity and that of the patient. Just when the Algerian people decided no longer to wait for others to treat them, colonialism prohibited the sale of medications and surgical instruments. Just when the Algerian was set to live and take care of himself, the occupying power doomed him to a horrible agony. Numerous families had to stand by, powerless, their hearts full of rancor, and watch the atrocious death by tetanus of wounded *moudjahidines* who had taken refuge in their houses. From the earliest months of the revolution, the directives of the National Front were clearly given: any wound, no matter how benign, automatically required an anti-tetanus vaccine injection. This the people knew. And when the wound, ugly to look at, had been cleaned of the dirt and grit picked up in the course of the retreat, the comrades of the wounded man would suddenly be seized with the fear of a tetanus infection. But the pharmacists were adamant: the sale of anti-tetanus vaccine was prohibited. Dozens and dozens of Algerians today can describe the slow, frighful death of a wounded man, progressively paralyzed, then twisted, and again paralyzed by the tetanus toxin. No one remains in the room to the end, they say in conclusion.

Yet the Algerian, when he sometimes would get a European to make his purchases, would see him return with the medicine which he had obtained without difficulty. The same Algerian had

previously begged all the pharmacists of the vicinity, and had finally given up, having felt the last pharmacist's hard and inquisitorial eye on him. The European would return, loaded down with medicines, relaxed, innocent. Such experiences have not made it easy for the Algerian to keep a balanced judgment toward members of the European minority. Science depoliticized, science in the service of man, is often nonexistent in the colonies. For this Algerian who for hours has begged unsuccessfully for a hundred grams of sterile cotton, the colonialist world constitutes a monolithic block. Alcohol being similarly prohibited, the wounds would be dressed with lukewarm water and, for lack of ether, amputations would be carried out without anaesthetics.

Now all these things that could not be found, that were held by the adversary, withdrawn from circulation, were to take on a new value. These medications, which were taken for granted before the struggle for liberation, were transformed into weapons. And the urban revolutionary cells having the responsibility for supplying medications were as important as those assigned to obtain information as to the plans and movements of the adversary. Even as the Algerian tradesman discovered ways of supplying the people with radios, so the Algerian pharmacist, the Algerian nurse, the Algerian doctor multiplied their efforts to make antibiotics and dressings available to the wounded at all times. From Tunisia and Morocco, finally, during the crucial months of 1956 and 1957, was to come a steady flow of medical supplies that saved an incalculable number of human lives.

The development of the war in Algeria, the setting up of units of the National Army of Liberation throughout the territory, brought about a dramatic public health problem. The increase in the number of areas constituting a threat to the adversary led him to interrupt regular activities, such as the visit of the doctor to the *douars*. From one day to the next, the population was left to fend for itself, and the National Liberation Front had to take drastic measures. It found itself faced with the necessity of setting up a system of public health capable of replacing the periodic visit of the colonial doctor. This is how the local cell member responsible for health became an important member of the revolutionary apparatus. The problem, moreover, became more and more

complex. Bombardments and raids on civilians were now added to natural diseases. It is a known fact that for one Algerian soldier hit, there are ten civilians killed or wounded. There is no lack of testimony from French soldiers to this effect. Under such circumstances, medical supplies and technicians became indispensable. It was during this period that orders were given to medical students, nurses, and doctors to join the combatants. Meetings were organized among political leaders and health technicians. After a short time, people's delegates assigned to handle public health problems came and joined each cell. All questions were dealt with in a remarkable spirit of revolutionary solidarity.

There was no paternalism; there was no timidity. On the contrary, a concerted effort was made to achieve the health plan that had been worked out. The health technician did not launch a "psychological approach program for the purpose of winning over the underdeveloped population." The problem was, under the direction of the national authority, to supervise the people's health, to protect the lives of our women, of our children, of our combatants.

We must dwell on the new reality that the rise of a national power has constituted in Algeria since 1954. This national authority has taken upon itself the responsibility for the health of the people, and the people have abandoned their old passivity. The people involved in this fight against death have shown exceptional conscientiousness and enthusiasm in their observance of the directives.

The Algerian doctor, the native doctor who, as we have seen, was looked upon before the national combat as an ambassador of the occupier, was reintegrated into the group. Sleeping on the ground with the men and women of the *mechtas*, living the drama of the people, the Algerian doctor became a part of the Algerian body. There was no longer that reticence, so constant during the period of unchallenged oppression. He was no longer "the" doctor, but "our" doctor, "our" technician.

The people henceforth demanded and practiced a technique stripped of its foreign characteristics. The war of liberation introduced medical technique and the native technician into the life of innumerable regions of Algeria. Populations accustomed to the

monthly or biennial visits of European doctors saw Algerian doctors settling permanently in their villages. The revolution and medicine manifested their presence simultaneously.

It is understandable that such facts should provide the basis for an incomparable dynamism and the point of departure for new attitudes. The problems of hygiene and of prevention of disease were approached in a remarkable creative atmosphere. The latrines recommended by the colonial administration had not been accepted in the *mechtas* but they were now installed in great numbers. Ideas on the transmission of intestinal parasites were immediately assimilated by the people. The elimination of stagnant pools was undertaken and the fight against postnatal ophthalmia achieved spectacular results. The problem was no longer that mothers neglected their children, but that aureomycin was at times unavailable. The people wanted to get well, wanted to care for themselves, and were anxious to understand the explanations proffered by fellow doctors or nurses.[8] Schools for nurses were opened and the illiterate, in a few days, proved capable of making intravenous injections.

Similarly, old superstitions began to crumble. Witchcraft, *maraboutism* (already considerably discredited as a result of the propaganda carried on by the intellectuals), belief in the *djinn*, all these things that seemed to be part of the very being of the Algerian, were swept away by the action and practice initiated by the revolution.[9] Even instructions difficult for highly technological societies to accept were assimilated by the Algerian. We shall give two significant examples of this.

First of all, a rule was made against giving a drink of water to a man wounded in the abdomen. Instructions were categorical. Lectures were given to the people. Not a boy, not a girl must be allowed to remain uninformed as to this rule: never a drop of water to a soldier wounded in the belly. After a battle, while awaiting the arrival of a doctor, the people gathered around the wounded would listen without weakening to the entreaties of the combatant. For hours, the women would obstinately refuse the wounded the requested swallow of water. And even the *moudjahid's* own son did not hesitate to say to his father, "Here is

your gun, kill me if you want, but I will not give you the water you ask for." When the doctor arrived, the necessary operation would be performed, and the *moudjahid* would have the maximum chance of recovering.

The second example relates to the strict diet to be followed in the course of a typhus infection. In the hospital the observance of the rules is obtained by the prohibition of family visits. For experience has shown that whenever a member of the family is allowed to visit the patient he lets himself be moved by the typhus patient's "hunger" and manages to leave him some cakes or some chicken. The result is that often an intestinal perforation results.

In the colonial situation, these things assume a special significance, for the colonized interprets this medical injunction as a new form of torture, of famine, a new manifestation of the occupant's inhuman methods. If the typhus patient is a child, one can understand the feelings that can overcome the mother. Out in the *djebel*, on the other hand, the Algerian nurse or doctor is able to win the patient's family over to a complete cooperation: hygienic precautions, regular administration of medications, prohibition of visits, isolation, and strict observance of diet for several days. The Algerian mother, who had never in her life seen a doctor, would follow the technician's instructions to the letter.

Specialists in basic health education should give careful thought to the new situations that develop in the course of a struggle for national liberation on the part of an underdeveloped people. Once the body of the nation begins to live again in a coherent and dynamic way, everything becomes possible. The notions about "native psychology" or of the "basic personality" are shown to be vain. The people who take their destiny into their own hands assimilate the most modern forms of technology at an extraordinary rate.

NOTES

1. French soldiers hospitalized in the psychiatric services of the French army in Algeria have all seen the experimental epileptic fits produced in Algerians and in infantrymen from south of the Sahara, for the

purpose of estimating the specific threshold of each of the different races. These men on whom the French doctors practiced these experiments were brought to the hospital on the "scientific pretext" of having to make further examinations.

It was left to the Algerian society alone, to the Algerian people alone, to manifest through combat its determination to put an end to such infamies, among others, on the national soil.

2. This particular observation is related to the overall attitude of the colonized who is hardly ever truthful before the colonizer. The colonized does not let on, does not confess himself, in the presence of the colonizer. The reader is referred to the communication before the 1955 Congress of French-Language Psychiatrists and Neurologists on "The Algerian and Avowal in Medico-Legal Practice."

3. There are obviously a certain number of doctors who act normally, who are human. But of them it will be said: "They are not like the others."

4. Medical practice in the colonies very often assumes an aspect of systematized piracy. Injections of twice-distilled water, billed as penicillin or vitamin B-12, chest X-rays, radiotherapy sessions "to stabilize a cancer," given by a doctor who has no radiological equipment, are examples. In the latter case, the doctor need only place the patient behind a sheet and after fifteen or twenty minutes announce that the session is over. It even happens that doctors in rural centers (several examples of this in Algeria are known) boast of taking x-rays with the aid of a vacuum cleaner. We may mention the case of a European doctor practicing in Rabelais (in the region of Orléansville) who explains how he manages, on market days, to earn more than 30,000 francs in the course of a morning. "I fill three syringes of unequal size with salt serum and I say to the patient, 'Which injection do you want, the 500, the 1000, or the 1500 franc one?' The patient," so the doctor explains, "almost always chooses the most expensive injection."

5. With respect to these measures the Council of the Order of Doctors in France adopted a very firm position consistent with the great French tradition.

Thus, its president, Professor Piedelièvre, in an official letter addressed to the Councils of the Order of Doctors of Algiers, of Constantine, and of Oran wrote: "May I remind you that in no case and under no pretext can professional secrecy be violated! I likewise point out to you that doctors are duty bound to treat all persons with the same conscientiousness, whatever be their religion or their race,

whether they are friends or enemies. I wish to draw your attention, finally, to the fact that the Code of Deontology, in its Article Three, has clearly stated: '*The doctor must treat all his patients with the same conscientiousness, whatever be their condition, their national-ity, their religion, their reputation and his feeling toward them.*'"
We may add further that many European doctors refused to apply the decisions adopted by the French authorities in Algeria.

6. H. Alleg, *La Question* (Paris: Editions de Minuit, 1958).
7. We have seen military doctors, called to the bedside of an Algerian soldier wounded in combat, refuse to treat him. The official pretext was that there was no longer a chance to save the wounded man. After the soldier had died, the doctor would admit that this solution had appeared to him preferable to a stay in prison where it would have been necessary to feed him while awaiting execution. The Algerians of the region of Blida know a certain hospital director who would kick the bleeding chests of the war wounded lying in the corridor of his establishment.
8. A change in attitude on the part of the Algerian toward the oc-cupier's hospital centers was likewise to be noted. It would in fact happen that the need of a particular medication or of a surgical operation impossible to carry out in the *maquis* would cause the doctor to advise the civilian to let himself be transferred to a hospital directed by the French. The hesitations and refusals that had been met with before the revolution vanished and the population would follow the orders given by the Algerian doctor in the *maquis*. This new attitude was very marked in 1956–57. I had occasion during this period to visit a great number of hospitals. The European doctors expressed their surprise to me at the time. Since the war, they said, "the Moslems let themselves be treated in the hospitals in the pro-portion of five to one as compared to the preceding years. One wonders why this is so." It should also be added that the hospital administrations in the *maquis* had a strategic interest in having civilians cared for by the French and keeping medical supplies for the soldiers, who could not be evacuated.
9. *Maraboutism*—the practice of medicine by the *marabout*, the Moslem priest. (Translator's note.)

   The *djinn* (plural *djnoun*) is a spirit. He haunts the houses and the fields. Popular belief attributed to him an important role in all the phenomena of life: birth, circumcision, marriage, sickness, death. In the case of disease, any impairment of health was interpreted as the work of a bad *djinn*.

E. RICHARD BROWN

PUBLIC HEALTH IN IMPERIALISM: EARLY ROCKEFELLER PROGRAMS AT HOME AND ABROAD

The professional public health field today owes much of its growth and development during the twentieth century to the needs of colonialism and neocolonialism. Imperialist powers were severely hampered by disease. Tropical diseases decimated the ranks of "mother country" personnel and reduced the efficiency of native populations as imperialism's workforce. As a writer in a popular journal observed in 1907:

> Disease still decimates native populations and sends men home from the tropics prematurely old and broken down. Until the white man has the key to the problem, this blot must remain. To bring large tracts of the globe under the white man's rule has a grandiloquent ring; but unless we have the means of improving the condition of the inhabitants, it is scarely more than an empty boast.[1]

To deal with this problem, to apply the medical sciences to the needs of imperialism, schools of tropical medicine were founded around the turn of the century. For example, Sir Patrick Manson organized the London School of Tropical Medicine in 1899 to help the Colonial Medical Service postpone the twilight of the British Empire.

These schools of tropical medicine, along with other medical research institutes, were largely successful in reducing the toll of tropical diseases, especially for European and American personnel. Whereas France's efforts to build a canal across the isthmus of Panama were thwarted by malaria and yellow fever, the efforts of Walter Reed, William Gorgas, and many other medical men made the subsequent U.S. attempt successful.

The Rockefeller public health philanthropies carried on the

imperialist tradition. Despite their humanitarian outward appearances, the major Rockefeller public health programs in the southern United States were intended to promote the economic development of the South as a regional economic, political, and cultural dependency of northern capital. Rockefeller Foundation public health programs in foreign countries were intended to help the United States develop and control the markets and resources of those nations.

These latter programs rested on four main propositions. First, U.S. control of the resources and markets, especially of nonindustrialized countries, was considered essential to the prosperity of this country. In addition, political control of such countries was considered important to maintaining their openness to profitable investment of "surplus" capital from the industrialized capitalist countries. Second, increased development of economically "backward" countries was seen as necessary to the successful exploitation of their resources, markets, and investment opportunities by capitalist countries. Third, tropical diseases—especially hookworm, malaria, and yellow fever—were believed to be obstacles to peoples of underdeveloped countries receiving the "benefits of civilization" and contributing to the economic development of their countries. And fourth, the foundation strategists believed that the biomedical sciences and their application through public health programs would increase the health and working capacity of these peoples *and* help induce them to accept Western industrial culture and U.S. economic and political domination.

By examining these programs—in particular, the Rockefeller Sanitary Commission for the Eradication of Hookworm Disease and the Rockefeller Foundation's International Health Commission—in the light of the other programs and interests of the foundations and their trustees and directors, we can see their connection to early twentieth century imperialism. We can also better understand the interests that led the Rockefeller philanthropies to help professionalize public health work, encouraging the formation of local public health departments, the hiring of full-time public health officers, and the funding of the first schools of public health in the United States, as well as others

abroad. The material for this paper was culled from the archives of the foundations—internal memos and correspondence—as well as from reports published by the foundations.

THE SOUTHERN U.S. "LAZY BUG"

The Rockefeller Sanitary Commission for the Eradication of Hookworm Disease was founded in 1909 with $1 million. In attempting to wipe out hookworm disease in the U.S. South, the program examined nearly 1.3 million persons in eleven southern states before it was merged with another Rockefeller program in 1914. It treated nearly 700,000 people for hookworm infection. It also helped to organize and rationalize state and county health departments in the South. While the program did not eradicate the disease, it did bring it under control in some areas, reduce its incidence, and (in some few locations) develop sufficient sanitation systems to halt the hookworm cycle and its spread.[2]

While these accomplishments are praiseworthy, the program carried other goals that were neither altruistic nor humanitarian. The Rockefeller Sanitary Commission was intended by its founders to integrate the "backward" South into the industrial economy controlled by northern capitalists. To that end, the commission sought to increase the productivity of southern agricultural and industrial workers.

By the time the Sanitary Commission was launched in 1909, John D. Rockefeller, Sr., his son Junior, and their chief lieutenant for their financial empire and philanthropies alike, Frederick T. Gates, already had seven years experience in the South.

The General Education Board, the first Rockefeller foundation, was formed in 1902 with an initial grant from Rockefeller, Sr., of $1 million.[3] It was formed out of a widespread continuing interest of northern industrialists and businessmen in promoting southern education as a means of expanding southern industrialization. As a 1902 memo from the General Education Board (GEB) hopefully noted, "The South with its varied resources and products has immense industrial potentialities, and its prosperous future will be assured with the right kind of education and training for its children of both races."

That meant vocational and business courses for white children, and vocational schools for blacks. The board believed "the Negro must be educated and trained, that he may be more sober, more industrious, more competent." The Rockefellers initially hoped the GEB would be a "vehicle through which capitalists of the North" could help build up southern schools, safely assured that their money would be spent efficiently and for the "right kind of education."

Soon after the secondary school development project started, the board began a systematic agricultural demonstration program throughout the South. Southern schools would train blacks as well as poor whites for industrial jobs in the "New South," and improved agricultural productivity would finance this development program and contribute to the country's exportable surplus. The GEB hired Seaman Knapp and spent nearly $1 million to bring Knapp's farm demonstration methods to southern farmers.[4] Knapp, who shared the imperialist views of his employers and the dominant capitalists of the time, boasted that "if we could teach the farmers who are now tilling the soil how to till it well—we should soon be able to buy any country that we take a fancy to."[5]

The Rockefeller efforts to expand southern agricultural productivity, and to prepare southern whites and blacks for industrialization in largely northern-owned mills and factories, were set back by the physical condition of the rural population. While involved in their school development and farm demonstration programs, the GEB officers "felt rather than knew that something else was the matter, that is, the people of the South were not as efficient as they ought to be."[6]

Charles Wardell Stiles, a government zoologist, convinced the Rockefeller philanthropists that the hookworm was "one of the most important diseases of the South" and a cause of "some of the proverbial laziness of the poorer classes of the white population." As the *New York Sun* publicized the discovery, they had found the "germ of laziness."[7]

It was no accident that the Rockefeller organization fixed on the hookworm for their first major venture into the public health field. In conditions of heavy infection the resulting disease in-

cludes a particularly debilitating anemia. According to J. M. May,[8] the anemia results from a combination of blood lost to the parasites and inadequate iron replacement through the diet. Hookworm anemia tends to be severe among people with low-protein and low-mineral diets. Thus hookworm disease, as distinguished from the mere invasion of the host by the parasites, is related to malnutrition, which especially affects workers on the bottom rungs of the social class structure.

Furthermore, the hookworm was (and is) widespread in areas of heavy investment by U.S. and European capital. Because the hookworm propagates itself in warm, moist climates, it is particularly associated with mining and the growing of rice, coffee, tea, sugar, cocoa, cotton, and bananas[9]—the resources and cash crops of concern to philanthropists who also have large investments in the South and underdeveloped tropical countries. Because hookworm disease reduced the strength and productivity of workers in these occupations, it had a direct effect on profits.

Whatever genuine pride the Rockefellers and Gates felt in relieving the suffering of thousands of southerners, their primary incentive was clearly the increased productivity of workers freed of the endemic parasite. Gates, the visionary of the Rockefeller health philanthropies, impressed upon the senior Rockefeller the dire economic consequences of the hookworm disease, using North Carolina as an example. The stocks of cotton mills located in the heavily infected tidewater counties were worth less than mills in other counties where fewer people were infected. "This is due," Gates explained, "to the inefficiency of labor in these cotton mills, and the inefficiency in the labor is due to the infection by the hookworm which weakens the operatives." Gates calculated that "It takes, by actual count, about twenty-five percent more laborers to secure the same results in the counties where the infection is heavier." It also took twenty-five percent more houses for the workers, more machinery, and thus more capital and higher operating costs. "This is why the stocks of such mills are lower and the profits lighter."[10]

The Rockefellers did not have any significant investment in southern textile mills. Rather, their extensive and widespread investments led them to a concern for the productivity of the

entire economy. And these financial interests made them broadly concerned with the social organization and institutions that could support or undermine their immensely profitable position in the United States. The Rockefellers, like their friend Andrew Carnegie, made their philanthropy an extension of their capital into the social superstructure. They fully understood the unity of their personal fortunes with the interests of the capitalist class as a whole, and they set about making educational institutions, the agricultural economy, and the public health more supportive of the new industrial order.

Although the hookworm campaign only partially fulfilled its objectives of reducing the economic and social burden of the disease, it did encourage (as intended) the creation of county public health departments staffed by full-time physicians charged with looking after the sanitation needs of the rural population. Thus the hookworm campaign and the Rockefellers' other southern programs were valuable to the generally poor people they reached. But they contributed at least as much to (a) encouraging the commercial organization of southern farming and placing local banks and the merchant class in control of the local southern agrarian economy, (b) cementing the position of blacks and poor whites as the agricultural and industrial laborers of the South, and (c) integrating the southern economy into the national dominion of northern capitalists.

PUBLIC HEALTH IN UNDERDEVELOPED COUNTRIES

As the five-year period initially designated for the Rockefeller Sanitary Commission came to a close, the work was taken up by the newly chartered Rockefeller Foundation.[11] The first act of the new foundation in 1913 was to create an International Health Commission to extend worldwide the hookworm and public health programs initiated in the United States. They placed a priority on the hookworm program "on account of the direct physical and economic benefits resulting from the eradication of the disease and also on account of the usefulness of this work as a means of creating and promoting influences."[12]

They immediately extended the hookworm programs abroad,

first to the nearby British Empire, then to Latin America and
Asia. In 1914 they began a campaign against yellow fever, and in
1915 another campaign against malaria.

These programs were undertaken in the context of the increasing importance of the United States in international financial and
industrial markets. In 1905 Gates, who was a Baptist minister
before he created the Rockefeller medical philanthropies, proclaimed the importance of missionaries to the economic prosperity of the United States. He urged Rockefeller, Sr., also a Baptist
and a frequent contributor to Baptist missionaries, to donate
$100,000 to an organization of Congregational mis-
sions. [13] "Now for the first time in the history of the world," Gates
explained to Rockefeller, "all the nations and all the islands of the
sea are actually open and offer a free field for the light and
philanthropy of the English speaking people. . . . Christian
agencies as a whole have very thoroughly invaded all coasts, all
strategic points, all ports of entry and are thoroughly intrenched
where they are." For Gates, transforming heathens into God-
fearing Christians was "no sort of measure" of the value of missionaries:

> Quite apart from the question of persons converted, the mere com-
> mercial results of missionary effort to our own land is worth, I had
> almost said a thousand fold every year of what is spent on mis-
> sions. . . . Missionary enterprise, viewed solely from a commercial
> standpoint, is immensely profitable. From the point of view of
> means of subsistence for Americans, our import trade, traceable
> mainly to the channels of intercourse opened up by missionaries, is
> enormous. Imports from heathen lands furnish us cheaply with
> many of the luxuries of life and not a few of the comforts, and with
> many things, indeed, which we now regard as necessities.

Advanced capitalism, however, required not only raw materials
and cheap products. It also needed new markets for its abundant
manufactured goods. As Gates added to Rockefeller's receptive
ear,

> Our imports are balanced by our exports to these same countries of
> American manufactures. Our export trade is growing by leaps and
> bounds. Such growth would have been utterly impossible but for the

commercial conquest of foreign lands under the lead of missionary endeavor. What a boon to home industry and manufacture!

The missionary effort in China was effective for a time in undermining Chinese self-determination. Missionaries were the velvet glove of imperialism frequently backed up by the mailed fist. Nevertheless, the missionary effort, promoted through schools and medical programs, was still a very transparent attempt to support European and American interests. As J. A. Hobson, an English economist, noted at the time, "Imperialism in the Far East is stripped nearly bare of all motives and methods save those of distinctively commercial origin."[14]

In China, as throughout the world, the Rockefeller philanthropists soon concluded that medicine and public health by themselves were far more effective than either missionaries or armies in pursuing the same ends. In China, the Rockefeller Foundation removed the Peking Union Medical College from missionary society control and established it under foundation direction. In China, the Philippines, Latin America, the West Indies, Ceylon and Malaya, Egypt, and other countries, the Rockefeller Foundation's International Health Commission organized, financed, and directed major campaigns against the hookworm.

These public health programs were blatantly intended, first, to raise the productivity of the workers in underdeveloped countries, second, to reduce the cultural autonomy of these agrarian peoples and make them amenable to being formed into an industrial workforce, and third, to assuage hostility to the United States and undermine goals of national economic and political independence.

INCREASING PRODUCTIVITY

In their public health programs conducted throughout the world, the Rockefellers and their staffs appear, from their own writings, to have been first and foremost concerned with the productivity of each country's labor force. The "efficiency" of plantation and mine workers was important, they noted, to ex-

tracting the produce and natural resources considered essential to U.S. prosperity. The hookworm reduced that efficiency. "It probably accounts, in very large degree," Gates wrote to Rockefeller, "for the character of tropical peoples."[15]

In virtually every annual report, every memorandum, and every discussion, the extent of hookworm infection was described and the loss in labor productivity estimated. Confirmation of the relationship was attested by increased productivity following treatment programs in each area.

The foundation officers were convinced of this relationship and impressed by the results of their campaign. A 1918 report on the "Economic Value of the Treatment of Hookworm Infection" demonstrated that for 320 laborers on two plantations in Costa Rica who were cured of hookworm infection, productivity increased dramatically.[16] One plantation increased its acreage under cultivation by nearly 50 percent—without the need of additional labor and at a smaller unit cost for cultivation. Each laborer was paid less per unit of work, but with increased strength was able to work harder and longer and "received more money in his pay envelope." The net results, concluded the report, "are happier, healthier, more *permanent* laborers producing more for themselves and for their employer."

Thus the Rockefeller Foundation's International Health Commission, and the Rockefeller Sanitary Commission before it, identified health as the capacity to work, and measured qualitative improvements in health by quantitative increases in productivity.

CULTURAL AND POLITICAL DOMINATION

The Rockefeller programs, however, did not concern themselves with workers' physical productivity alone. They were also intended to reduce the cultural resistance of "backward" and "uncivilized" peoples to the domination of their lives and societies by industrial capitalism. Whether in the jungles of Latin America or the isolated islands of the Philippines, the Rockefeller Foundation discovered what the missionaries before them under-

stood: that medicine was an almost irresistible force in the colonization of nonindustrialized countries.

In the Philippines, the foundation outfitted a hospital ship to bring medical care and the "benefits of civilization" to rebellious Moro tribesmen. Foundation officers were ecstatic that such medical work made it "possible for the doctor and nurse to go in safety to many places which it has been extremely dangerous for the soldier to approach." Their medical work paved "the way for establishing industrial and regular schools." In the words of foundation president George Vincent, "Dispensaries and physicians have of late been peacefully penetrating areas of the Philippine Islands and demonstrating the fact that for purposes of placating primitive and suspicious peoples *medicine has some advantages over machine guns.*"[17]

Finally, the Rockefeller Foundation hoped these programs would facilitate U.S. control over the economies and political institutions of the host countries. Despite many public relations statements that "A constant aim of the International Health Board is to turn over to government agencies, public health activities which have been demonstrated to be effective,"[18] in reality the foundation was quite determined to keep control of the programs in their own hands. In Latin America, as elsewhere, they created organizations and goverment ministries and departments that ensured that "the *entire* control of *all* the *money* would be held by our people and not the natives."[19]

The foundation desired direct control over these health programs for two reasons. First, the end result—increased productivity—was so important to them that they did not want the reputedly inefficient indigenous people or their corrupt local and national political rulers making a mess of things. They hired some native doctors and trained local personnel who were willing to cooperate with the foundation to run programs "efficiently." Throughout its worldwide operation the foundation seemed willing to turn programs over only to British colonial governments and other governments that would keep the personnel selected and trained by the foundation.

Furthermore, the indigenous governments were seen largely as

vehicles for a penetrating political, economic, and cultural control by U.S. corporations and agencies. In China, for example, the Rockefeller Foundation's Peking Union Medical College was conducted entirely by their own staff from New York and a local office in Peking. In 1920 the PUMC resident director, Roger Greene, urged foundation officers in New York to get U.S. bankers to offer a major loan to the Chinese government for famine relief. His motives were perhaps humanitarian, but with a heavy overlay of expediency as well. "I believe," he wrote,

> that the Chinese government would for this special purpose accept a very large degree of foreign control of expenditure. The practical experience gained under the operation of such a loan might be of enormous value in creating a better understanding between the bankers and the Chinese government. [20]

The end goal of this control and of the native population's "experience" with U.S.-directed health programs was to establish in the hearts and minds of the peoples of the recipient countries a more favorable attitude toward *continued* U.S. economic and political domination. While business interests had taken the lead in establishing "closer relations" with Latin America, business is "necessarily more interested in what it can get out of South America than what it has to give." Because of the humanitarian character of the public health programs, however, Rockefeller Foundation officers understood that "the byproducts of our work in the form of friendly international relations might be even more important than the relief and control of [hookworm] or yellow fever." [21]

Many prominent Latin Americans accepted the intended public image of the foundation. In Costa Rica, the Catholic curate, Father Lombardo, told a public conference:

> You all know we never cared for or trusted the Yankees, but since this institution has come and worked here, and is showing us that they [the Yankees] have some heart in them, we feel like giving them the embrace of brotherhood and making them feel more welcome hereafter. I should love to shake Mr. Rockefeller's hand and say: "You are one of us." [22]

Other Latin Americans were not so gullible. A prominent Nicaraguan lawyer called the Rockefeller public health programs "one of the many 'advance guards' of the American conquest."[23]

By the early 1920s the Rockefeller Foundation officers concluded that in less than a decade of work with more than sixty countries, "We have seen an attitude of cold curiosity as to what our real motives might be, give place to an implicit trust which opens all doors."[24]

SCHOOLS OF PUBLIC HEALTH

The importance of these programs and the lack of sufficient trained personnel led the Rockefeller Foundation officers to promote the development of schools of public health. The foundation's International Health Commission badly needed trained staff for its worldwide attacks on hookworm, malaria, and yellow fever. It also needed a continuing supply of public health professionals to meet the demands for trained personnel at local and state levels generated by the hookworm campaign.

Thus the Rockefeller Foundation became the first major source of funds for professional education in public health. Largely because of their great trust in William H. Welch's commitment to scientific and technical approaches to health issues, the Rockefeller Foundation gave $1 million to The Johns Hopkins University between 1916 and 1922 to organize the first full-fledged school of public health in the United States. Between 1921 and 1927 they gave $3.5 million to Harvard University to organize a second school. In all, they contributed more than $25 million for the development of public health schools in the United States and abroad. They also spent several millions more on fellowships for foreign medical personnel to be trained in public health sciences.[25]

Just as the European powers had created schools of tropical medicine to provide scientific medical knowledge and specially trained physicians for their colonial empires, the Rockefeller Foundation wanted its schools to develop useful medical knowledge and train personnel for the programs and departments it was

helping to organize. The Rockefeller philanthropies thus contributed directly and indirectly to the development of the public health profession.

DISCUSSION

Obviously the Rockefeller Foundation programs were a mixed bag. To the extent that they improved the health of indigenous populations, they were beneficial to those peoples. To the extent that they fostered greater economic and political control and profit by European and U.S. capitalist nations, they were insidious forces that worked to the detriment of the peoples they were ostensibly helping.

These consequences were neither minor nor incidental. Clothed in the ideological justifications prevalent in the period—as Gates put it, "Our improved methods of production and agriculture, manufacture and commerce, our better social and political institutions, our better literature, philosophy, science, art, refinement, morality and religion"[26]—both public health programs in recipient countries and corporate profits derived from these countries were seen as beneficent transplantings of Western civilization. Health was defined as the capacity to work, and increased productivity of populations was the measure of success of public health programs.

Although foundation programs were often closely linked to Rockefeller investments—for example, major medical education programs were begun in China and Turkey corresponding to major marketing operations of the Standard Oil Company— much of their work reflected a broad view of the needs of U.S. capitalism. Gates and contemporary anti-imperialist writers Hobson[27] and Lenin[28] agreed that advanced capitalism *requires* the economic conquering of foreign markets, natural resources, and opportunities for profitable investment of "mother country" capital. As manufactured products and capital alike filled the most profitable domestic markets in the late nineteenth century, the increasingly monopolistic industrialists and financiers sought new and more profitable outlets. As we have seen, the link between

the Rockefeller Foundation health programs and the needs of imperialism were well understood and intended by the Rockefellers and Gates.

Once these programs were launched by the foundation's top officers, the internal logic and historical conditions assured that the imperialist ends would be served even if mid-level officers, field directors, and professional personnel did not consciously promote imperialism through their programs. First, the programs had a logic and momentum of their own. Acceptance of European and American medical theories and practice implied submission to the authority and superiority of these foreign cultures. Incorporating modern technology, medical and public health programs were correctly seen by the foundation officers as undermining the resistance of agrarian and traditional peoples to "industrialization"—that is, to their exploitation as productive labor in the mines, plantations, and factories owned by European and American capitalists. As Frantz Fanon pointed out, colonized people also viewed Western medicine as inseparable from colonization.[29] In the social psychology of imperialism, to submit to the Rockefeller health programs was to submit to Rockefeller and American cultural, political, and—underlying it all—economic domination. One could feel good working in or supporting the humanitarian public health programs and ignore the dominating consequences of these programs that operated whether one was conscious of the dynamic or not.

Furthermore, the historical reality coincided with the social perceptions of the Rockefeller philanthropists and the colonized. Then, as now, development capital was overwhelmingly possessed and tightly controlled by the advanced capitalist nations, eager to export their capital for the higher rates of return usually available in underdeveloped countries. Industrialization, promoted by health programs as well as by political and economic policies, required outside capital, and the few countries able to export capital were in a position to "help." Thus even if unintended by Gates and Rockefeller, the foundation's public health programs would have contributed indirectly but significantly to the economic exploitation of the underdeveloped world by the

advanced capitalist nations. No conspiracy was needed to assure that these ostensibly humanitarian programs served the needs of imperialism.

Finally, the great foundations are inextricably tied to imperialism. Their wealth came from the giant financial and industrial corporations associated with the rise of imperialism. They are run by trustees and officers who, by their material interests and ideological commitments, are part of the corporate capitalist class.

The health professionals who worked in these programs did not own or control the corporations that profited from foreign trade and investments, but they did share the material advantages that accrued to the "mother country." And they certainly shared the racist and ethnocentric ideologies that justify imperialism. Welch, the first dean of The Johns Hopkins Medical School and its School of Hygiene and Public Health, praised the facilitating role of medical science in European and American "efforts to colonize and to reclaim for civilization (sic) vast tropical regions."[30] Just as missionaries saw themselves promoting Christian civilization in their work, so too did public health professionals join foundation programs to bring the "benefits of civilization" to "backward" peoples through their medical work.

Public health programs have been the humanitarian partner of American imperialism for more than sixty years. In 1954 John C. McClintock, an assistant vice-president of United Fruit, neatly summed up the relationship between health and profits that has been a concern of these programs in the tropics:

> In the underdeveloped areas where American companies have gone, where they have brought great enterprises into fruition, where they are continuing, one of the primary factors was to establish conditions of health where people could not only exist but also could work.[31]

Public health programs were undertaken in tropical countries, he continued, "because they could not get out the ore, or raise the bananas, or pump the oil unless these fundamentals were taken care of."

While many professionals in the field may have been only dimly aware of the supportive role they were playing for imperialism, certainly many were and are quite conscious of it. In 1962 the National Academy of Sciences–National Research Council issued a report on tropical health, supported by the U.S. Army, the National Institutes of Health, and the Rockefeller Foundation.[32] In a chapter on "Tropical Health and the Economy of the United States," the authors, sounding very much like Frederick T. Gates writing about missionaries a half century earlier, observed that with the increasingly important role of foreign trade and investments, particularly in Latin America, Arica, and Asia, the health of tropical peoples is of material importance to the U.S. economy. "There is no doubt," they concluded, "that a reduction in debilitating infectious diseases and improvements in diet will increase the capacity of tropical populations for work and represent an economic contribution to the welfare of the nation." In testifying to the importance of tropical health, the authors approvingly quote economist Stacy May who called tropical medicine the "midwife of economic progress in the underdeveloped areas of the world." For many years a director of IBEC (a Rockefeller-controlled investment corporation), May argued that, "Where mass diseases are brought under control, productivity tends to increase—through increasing the percentage of adult workers as a proportion of the total population, [and] through augmenting their strength and ambition to work."

CONCLUSION

There is certainly nothing inherently evil in increasing productivity by improving people's health. When such measures enrich the lives of the recipient peoples and enable them to develop their own countries in ways they determine to be in their best interests, such health programs are very much humanitarian. The Rockefeller Foundation programs, however, were only secondarily concerned with the interests of the native populations. Their primary goals were to enrich plantation, mine, and factory own-

ers and ultimately foreign imperialist powers—or in the case of the American South, the largely northern capitalist class. In a clear example of ideological thinking, the interests of the native populations were assumed to be identical to the interests of American corporations.

Thus, these programs were *not* devoid of politics. By their definition of health as the capacity to work, by their technological content that weakened traditional and agrarian cultural autonomy, by historical conditions that assured that economic development (when unfettered by national independence struggles) would profit foreign capitalist classes, and by their undermining of forces seeking economic and political independence, the Rockefeller public health programs were loaded with political and economic values and consequences.

Ostensibly humanitarian public health programs may, as we have seen, carry oppressive consequences, whether intended or not. It is incumbent on health professionals and their associations to include in their concerns not only technical competence but also the political, economic, and social ends of programs in their field. We may examine the material interests that underlie all public health programs, whether sponsored by the Rockefeller Foundation, the U.S. Agency for International Development, or the World Health Organization. It is certainly easier to do so retrospectively with the aid of internal files, as I have done with the Rockefeller programs. Nevertheless, such analysis may make it more difficult for the positive values of health work to blind us to its related dangers. If public health is to be an advocate of the interests of the majorities of all peoples, it must not be used to dominate and oppress them.

NOTES

1. G. E. M. Vaughan, "A School of Tropical Medicine," *The World's Work* 14 (1907): 8898–901.
2. G. Williams, *The Plague Killers* (New York: Charles Scribner's Sons, 1969); M. Boccaccio, "Ground Itch and Dew Poison: The Rockefeller Sanitary Commission, 1909–1914," *J. Hist. Med. and Allied Sciences* 27 (1972): 30–53; J. H. Cassedy, "The 'Germ of Laziness' in the

South, 1900–1915: Charles Wardell Stiles and the Progressive Paradox," *Bull. Hist. Med.* 45 (1971): 159–69.

3. R. B. Fosdick, *Adventure in Giving: The Story of the General Education Board* (New York: Harper & Row, 1962).

4. Ibid.

5. W. H. Page, "Teaching Farmers to Farm," *The World's Work* 14 (1907): 8987–989.

6. W. Buttrick, "Notes from the Old Man Buttrick," General Education Board files, Rockefeller Foundation Archives (1924).

7. Williams, *The Plague Killers*.

8. J. M. May, *The Ecology of Human Disease* (New York: MD Publications, 1958).

9. Ibid.

10. F. T. Gates to J. D. Rockefeller, December 12, 1910, Record Group 2, Rockefeller Family Archives.

11. Williams, *The Plague Killers*; R. B. Fosdick, *The Story of the Rockefeller Foundation* (New York: Harper, 1952).

12. Rockefeller Foundation, Minutes, May 22, 1913, Rockefeller Foundation Archives.

13. F. T. Gates to J. D. Rockefeller, January 31, 1905, Letterbook No. 350, Record Group 1, Rockefeller Family Archives.

14. J. A. Hobson, *Imperialism* (1902; London: George Allen and Unwin, 1938).

15. F. T. Gates to J. D. Rockefeller, June 30, 1911, Record Group 2, Rockefeller Family Archives.

16. G. C. Cox, "Economic Value of the Treatment of Hookworm Infection in Costa Rica," International Health Commission files, Rockefeller Foundation Archives.

17. G. E. Vincent, *The Rockefeller Foundation—A Review of Its War Work, Public Health Activities, and Medical Examination Projects in 1917* (New York: Rockefeller Foundation, 1918); and "Hospital Ship for Sulu Archipelago," *The Rockefeller Foundation* 1, nos. 13–14 (1916).

18. Rockefeller Foundation, Annual Report (New York, 1918).

19. J. H. White to W. Rose, August 14, 1915, and W. Rose to J. H. White, August 17, 1915, International Health Commission files, Rockefeller Foundation Archives.

20. R. S. Greene to J. D. Greene, November 5, 1920, China Medical Board files, Rockefeller Foundation Archives.

21. W. Rose, "Committee to Study and Report on Medical Conditions and Progress in Brazil," October 26, 1915, Medical Education in

Brazil, International Health Commission files, Rockefeller Foundation Archives.

22. Quoted in W. Rose to S. J. Murphy, June 23, 1916, Record Group 2, Rockefeller Family Archives.

23. Quoted in C. Lewerth, "Source Book for a History of the Rockefeller Foundation," p. 481, Rockefeller Foundation Archives.

24. W. Rose to J. D. Rockefeller, Jr., August 3, 1921, Record Group 2, Rockefeller Family Archives.

25. Williams, *The Plague Killers*; Fosdick, *The Story of the Rockefeller Foundation*.

26. F. T. Gates to J. D. Rockefeller, February 2, 1905, Letterbook No. 350, Record Group 1, Rockefeller Family Archives.

27. Hobson, *Imperialism*.

28. V. I. Lenin, *Imperialism—The Highest Stage of Capitalism* (New York: International Publishers, 1939).

29. F. Fanon, "Medicine and Colonialism," in F. Fanon, *Studies in a Dying Colonialism* (New York: Grove Press, 1967). Reprinted in this volume.

30. W. H. Welch, "The Benefits of the Endowment of Medical Research," in *Addresses Delivered at the Opening of the Laboratories in New York City, May 11, 1906* (New York: Rockefeller Institute for Medical Research, 1906).

31. Industrial Council for Tropical Health and Harvard School of Public Health, *Industry and Tropical Health II*, Proceedings of the Second Conference, New York and Boston, April 20–22, 1954.

32. *Tropical Health—A Report on a Study of Needs and Resources*, National Academy of Sciences–National Research Council, Publication No. 996 (Washington, D.C., 1962).

JAMES A. PAUL

MEDICINE AND IMPERIALISM

The accumulation of capital and the accompanying drive to maximize profit are the basic organizing principles of the medical system in capitalist society. It is evident that this entails profitable markets for drugs, medical equipment, and service industries as well as markets for financial services and health facilities construction. It is less understood that organized medicine helps to establish and maintain the capitalist system itself. Yet medicine clearly works to reinforce class differences through sharply differential provision of services. It also engages in propaganda, intelligence collection, and socialization to the main forms of capitalist rule and domination. An examination of medical science and medical policy must, therefore, raise the broadest questions of social and political power: the general movement toward the accumulation and centralization of capital as well as the development and mutual antagonism of social classes and the struggle over the dominant ideological system.

We will examine capitalist medicine in the context of imperialism. By imperialism we mean foreign expansion and conquest associated with the growth of monopoly in the major capitalist countries. This process dates from the "classic" period of late nineteenth century colonialism. It continues through the neocolonialism of the present epoch, for the interests of a handful of imperialist metropolitan centers have never ceased to dominate the political economy of much of the rest of the world.[1] Imperialism is an excellent vantage point from which to see the social and political functions of medicine. In the impoverishment, plunder, and violence of the colonies and neocolonies,

capitalist social relations assume their most transparent and clearly identifiable image. Medicine has from the beginning functioned in the service of imperialism, supporting logically the voracious search for ever wider markets and profitable deals.

Our analysis necessarily makes a distinction between medicine and health. By health we mean a general life condition characterized by physical, mental, and social well-being and not merely the absence of disease.[2] By medicine we mean the science and social organization developed in the advanced capitalist countries primarily for the treatment of physical infirmity. This distinction permits us to inquire how medicine impairs health as well as how it promotes health. It also permits us to examine more clearly the ideological character of medical science. We can see, for instance, how medicine appropriates the social definition of health in a narrow sense, thus obscuring the broader health-destroying effects of the social order it supports. We can also see how medical science, rather than eliminate the social roots of ill-health, promotes a commodity-based disease therapy. And finally, we can better grasp the role of the doctor, not as benevolent practitioner of universal science but as purveyor of capitalist values and as enthusiastic agent of imperial rule.

We draw upon research on medicine and French imperialism in Morocco during the past century, as well as contemporary examples of medicine and American imperialism.[3] After a brief examination of health in an imperialist setting, we consider five principal features of medical-imperial politics: (1) physicians as covert diplomats, (2) physicians as propagandists and spies among the colonial peoples, (3) medicine as a vehicle for imperialist propaganda in the metropolitan center, (4) colonies as territories for medical sales and medical experimentation, and (5) medicine as a vehicle for establishing and maintaining exploitative social relations. In conclusion, we note some principal contradictions of imperialist medicine.

IMPERIALISM AND HEALTH

Colonial conquest brought medicine to vast areas of the world. This does not mean that it simply introduced health to the "hea-

then," though there are definite health achievements to its credit. In Morocco, French colonial medicine introduced field medical stations and mobile medical teams which delivered care to many remote areas. It prompted mass sprayings and inoculations to prevent the worst communicable diseases. French medical scientists developed new methods for the prevention and treatment of tuberculosis, typhus, and trachoma. But the health of the Moroccan people did not gain substantially from the imperial relationship. Conquering colonial armies killed more than 100,000 Moroccans and injured or maimed several times that number; casualties amounted to more than 5 percent of the total population. French troops destroyed whole villages, burned crops, and killed livestock. They razed mosques and schools. The war of pacification lasted twenty-five years.

Settler farmers and metropolitan companies, backed by the French army, seized a million hectares of the richest land from the Moroccan peasantry. About a sixth of all food-producing land was thus diverted from local subsistence farming to the production of cash crops for export—first wheat, later wine and citrus. As a result, Moroccan food consumption fell substantially. Since grazing lands were reduced, Moroccan meat consumption declined: from over three meals of meat per week in the 1880s to only one meal per week eighty years later. Grain consumption decreased also, while the use of unhealthful sugar and tea (imported by French companies) grew substantially. The overall drop in caloric intake, joined to more strenuous wage labor in colonial field and factory, increased the incidence of malnutrition, thus lowering disease resistance. Plague and cholera swept the malnourished and weakened population, taking thousands of lives. Tuberculosis and syphilis ravaged slum-dwelling urban migrants, while the dilapidated native hospitals could not begin to serve even the worst cases. In addition, some 40,000 Moroccans either died or were injured while serving in the French army in two world wars and numerous colonial conflicts from West Africa to Indochina. Countless other Moroccans were maimed or killed in French-owned factories, fields, and mines. Medicine did not *cause* these health atrocities, of course, but, as we shall see, it supported them, participated in them, and apologized for them.

Such is the context in which we must evaluate the record of French imperialist medicine.

Now, the United States dispatches its doctors along with soldiers and business agents to a worldwide network of dependent underdeveloped countries. American medical aid to these regimes, amounting to more than $1 billion in the past decade,[4] has certainly achieved its successes, including the spectacular eradication of smallpox. But the fundamentally unhealthful side of imperialism persists. Recent U.S.-sponsored wars, counterrevolutions, and pacification programs have spread death and havoc in southern Africa, South and Central America, Southeast Asia, and the Middle East. Six million dead and 10 million refugees are the minimum toll in Indochina; among civilians in South Vietnam alone, war claimed 1.5 million casualties, including nearly half a million dead, 40,000 amputees, 20,000 brain injured, 30,000 blind, and 10,000 paraplegics.[5] A million Indonesians were slaughtered in the fierce anti-Communist crusade in 1965. Tens of thousands have been killed, tortured, mutilated, and jailed in continuing campaigns in Guatemala and Chile.[6]

Widespread hunger and starvation have resulted from the operations of American agribusiness, which removes land from local food production to raise bananas, coffee, cocoa, peanuts, cotton, jute, rubber, and other export crops. Famines now sweeping Africa and Asia are largely due to this diversion of local resources and the accompanying soil depletion of rapacious one-crop farming.[7] Many similar causes of morbidity suggest themselves, not least the rampant heroin traffic, directly sponsored by CIA pacification programs.[8] Clearly, imperialism is not a healthful social arrangement. Let us now turn to see how medicine has contributed to the establishment and development of this health-destructive system.

MEDICINE AND DIPLOMACY

European physicians frequently participated in the diplomacy of colonial conquest. Their medical training and practice imbued them with a firm belief in the benevolence and universality of

medical science, and by extension European "civilization" more generally. It was but a short step from doctor-knows-best paternalism to the advocacy of the imperialist "civilizing mission" and "white man's burden." Many doctors, therefore, accepted covert diplomatic assignments, using their professional role as an effective cover. France used doctors in this way in its intensive effort to seize Morocco as a colony. Its competitors—Britain, Spain, and Germany—did the same.

European chancelleries employed physicians directly as diplomatic agents. These doctors, often trained in earlier colonial service, carried out their tasks with skill and audacity, insinuating themselves into favor with the reigning sultan, his wives and family members, or other important political persons. Taking advantage of their miraculous cures and their position of professional confidence, they established contacts where more ordinary diplomatic methods failed. They argued subtly for favorable treaties, arranged contracts for metropolitan manufacturers, gained mining concessions, promoted bank loans, passed along intimate intelligence concerning the affairs of state, and sowed intrigue and discord when this suited their larger diplomatic purposes.

Dr. Fernand Linarès, an army doctor working in concert with the French foreign service, was the principal foreign diplomatic figure at the Moroccan court for more than a quarter century—from the early 1870s until 1900. As one French ambassador described him, Linarès was a "precious liaison with the [government], capable of neutralizing rival influences . . . and preparing the way for what is called 'the peaceful penetration' of Morocco."[9] A score of European doctors were active in similar missions in Morocco in this period. Their medical activities were totally subsumed by their political mission, since they undertook only such healing as diplomacy required. Their main job was to help impose colonial control over independent Morocco.

Even after Moroccan independence in 1956, France continued to place medico-diplomatic intermediaries with persons in power. One such figure was Dr. Henri Dubois-Roquebert, personal surgeon and confidant of King Mohammed V. He negotiated to protect French business interests during the transition to an

independent regime and continued to practice the diplomatic arts until his death only three years ago.

The United States has used medical diplomats in much the same fashion. Dr. Kevin Cahill, an American Public Health Service doctor who served in West Africa in the early 1960s, has written of his "intimate contact with numerous diplomatic efforts" as physician to prime ministers and other government leaders. He claims he continuously influenced policy during changing regimes and was a conduit for "highly confidential messages" between American and African officials. Reflecting the imperial tradition of Linarès and Dubois-Roquebert, Cahill concludes that "combining medicine and diplomacy represents a most natural vehicle for modern international communication."[10]

MEDICINE, MASS PROPAGANDA, AND ESPIONAGE IN THE COLONIES

Beyond the court intrigues of high diplomacy, the foreign services and armed forces of the major metropolitan powers used doctors as spies and propagandists among the native masses. The same medical-ideological perspectives and the same professional cover which made doctors enthusiastic and effective diplomats made them fitting agents for this type of work as well.

In Morocco, British doctors penetrated the interior around 1880, sponsored by Presbyterian missionary societies. Winning few converts, they nevertheless raised the prestige of Britain by their medical miracles and they sent home useful intelligence reports. The French and Germans then sent their own contingents of doctors—known as "foreign affairs missionaries"—to combat the British offensive. These secular missionaries were usually army doctors on loan to the foreign service. Like their religious counterparts, they used medical skills to gain access to remote and resistant elements of the Moroccan population. They sowed discontent among groups and tribes and conducted standard military intelligence: gathering strategic information on the military organization and defenses, carrying out political and social research, and preparing maps for pending colonial invasion.

Later, doctors played a part in the French conquest and pacification of Morocco. General Lyautey sent specially constituted mobile medical units in the vanguard of the invading armies in 1907. These units provided medical care to the enemy tribesmen. The army physicians spoke to local leaders during their medical consultations, offering a choice of continued benevolent care or certain death and destruction. This tactic won the French numerous victories without battle (though it did not prevent a long resistance). Army physicians also joined intelligence officers on scouting forays. They offered medical care to Moroccans in exchange for information on local terrain, tribal defenses, and the like. Such military work continued throughout the twenty-five years of pacification. In fact, during the remainder of the colonial period and beyond, the Moroccan public health service retained a military character and a perspective rooted in the early pacification concerns.

American foreign policy has put medicine to similar uses. In 1966, U.S. Special Forces psychiatrist Leonard Friedman argued that the "mutual trust" developed through medical programs would contribute to the "solution of the South Vietnamese insurgency."[11] "Medical Civic Action," in fact, assumed a major place in U.S. pacification plans, with wholehearted support from the U.S. medical community, including the AMA, Dr. John Knowles, and Surgeon-General Leonard Heaton. In 1968, when Col. Spurgeon Neel reviewed the results in *Military Medicine*, he concluded that medicine was indeed effective as an "apolitical avenue through which favorable influence may be maintained."[12] Congressman Hugh Carey wrote in the same vein in 1971 about "The War We *Can* Win." Suggesting that U.S. overseas health programs should be expanded, he cited medical counterinsurgency successes in Vietnam as well as in Latin America as proof of the value of medicine as an American foreign policy weapon in an increasingly hostile world.[13]

MEDICINE AND IMPERIALIST PROPAGANDA ON THE HOME FRONT

In order to win mass support at home, imperialism has always cloaked with moral justifications its underlying drive for accumulation and profit. Medicine has contributed significantly to this

propaganda, particularly through the unquestioned authority of the doctor. Doctors have not hesitated to diagnose the ills of the most backward lands and prescribe a strong dose of "assistance." They have thus helped convince the metropolitan working class to accept the cost of imperial ventures and to see as virtuous sacrifice the payment of special taxes and enrollment in fresh army levies.

During the precolonial penetration of Morocco, European physicians lobbied and wrote in favor of colonial takeover. They described the bad health conditions in Morocco and the great contribution European medicine had made to improving native health. Only under colonialism, they argued, could the full benefits of European medical science be made available to the native masses. By describing primitive and superstitious traditional health practices, they reinforced the view that Moroccans were savage, ignorant, fanatic, and unable to manage their own affairs. This medical argumentation gained wide circulation and popularity, helping to form mass opinion in favor of colonial rule. So powerful was the effect of medical propaganda that the French government used it as the immediate justification for armed intervention. When an angry mob in Marrakesh murdered Dr. Emile Mauchamp, a notorious French spy, the metropolitan press responded with outrage and indignation. In fact, French troops were already crossing the border from Algeria. The colonial conquest of Morocco had begun.

Throughout the colonial period and even thereafter, medicine continued to serve as an important justification of French involvement in Morocco. One colonial panegyrist spoke of physicians as "apostles" of colonialism who "ennobled" the entire colonial enterprise. Few colonial apologias did not give pride of place to medical accomplishments. The doctors themselves wrote many books and articles celebrating their kindly deeds, their contribution to "peaceful pacification," and their inspiration of boundless native gratitude.

Medical propaganda on the home front has been used to justify American imperialism as well. Dr. Tom Dooley, the hospital ship "Hope," and other symbols of American humanitarianism have been widely publicized as examples of the benign character of

American overseas interests. Such medical propaganda was extensively used to counter criticisms of the American war in Vietnam. Dr. Howard Rusk, the *New York Times* medical editor, systematically obscured the war's devastating effects by lauding the medical assistance programs. In 1966, he wrote that "Vietnam has a long way to go before its complex health problems are solved, but it has also gone a long way in moving toward their solution during the last year."[14] In 1967, President Johnson requested AMA vice-president F. J. L. Blasingame and a "distinguished team" of physicians to investigate Vietnamese health conditions. Among other things, the team managed to conclude that it was not American napalm bombs that caused the many petroleum burns suffered by Vietnamese civilians but rather a "careless use of gasoline in stoves not intended for this purpose."[15] Even in the final hours, U.S. policy makers masked their war plans with a medical cover, emphasizing the medical-humanitarian aspect of the massive aid by which they hoped to shore up the beleaguered Thieu regime.

MEDICAL SALES AND MEDICAL EXPERIMENTATION

When European medicine entered the colonial areas, some standard metropolitan practices were modified. Nonetheless, colonial medicine did not deviate far from the European model. It remained a hospital-centered, curative system, using large quantities of manufactured goods such as pills, serums, powders, dressings, hospital equipment, and medical vehicles. Medicine thus expanded markets and raised the profits of firms that produced or shipped medical products. This process was evident in Morocco as commodity-centered medicine spread relentlessly and medical imports soared. Hastening the process were legal restrictions on traditional medical practice as well as disruption of the traditional urban hygiene based on baths, sunny courtyards, and pure water fountains.

Further medical profits flowed from hospital construction programs which favored colonial contractors and cement producers. The big banks and insurance companies profitably placed the hospital construction loans and administered medical insurance

programs. Since Morocco's economy was dominated by a half-dozen bank holding companies, the profits realized in the medical sphere cannot be considered in isolation. They constituted but one part of the enormous gains reaped by these interests from the whole Moroccan economy. Colonial medicine, colonial agriculture, colonial mining, and colonial manufacturing were thus developed by a single nexus of interest, for a single purpose.

Pharmaceutical manufacturers have drawn a special advantage from imperialism. They have used the colonial populations as subjects for drug tests without taking the expensive precautions generally necessary in the metropolis. Drug experimentation in Morocco led to a new typhus vaccination and to aureomycin pommade for eye disease. But such experiments were not always directed at the health needs of Moroccans. Carried out in a careless manner, they frequently damaged the health of the subject population.

American medicine is similarly product-centered and curative. U.S. government programs have fostered this type of medicine through medical "aid," stimulating sales not only for pharmaceuticals but also for the most expensive types of hospital and research equipment: electron microscopes, radiation treatment machines, laser beam surgery equipment, and similar products of the latest medical technology.[16] Nor have U.S. policy makers failed to emulate their European cousins in a predilection for medical experimentation. One notorious case has been the testing of harmful birth control products. American medical teams have carried out such research in dozens of underdeveloped countries, including Puerto Rico, Honduras, Brazil, and India. Death, birth defects, and widespread involuntary sterility have resulted from these callous efforts at cheap product development.[17]

MEDICINE AND SOCIAL RELATIONS

The medical system helps create new social relations, fostering the spread of capitalism at the expense of primitive social modes. In particular, it contributes to the transformation of peasant agriculturalists into colonial wage laborers. At the hospital or

health station, many peasants experience for the first time a rationalized bureaucratic organization of the capitalist type. They learn to adapt to its methods of operation, developing such skills and attitudes as punctuality, discipline, and deference to authorities of the central state. They also learn that money wages purchase the best care and that the main centers for medical treatment are far away in the great colonial cities. In this way, the peasantry are encouraged to abandon the old ways of traditional society. The cities beckon; hopes of what wages may buy are nourished. When life on the land finally becomes impossible, the peasants are ready to enter the harsh new world of exploitation which the colonial wage system offers them.

Medicine also helps create a new social layer of professionals who mediate between the native masses and the colonial property owners. During the early phase of the colonial period, entry into these professions is practically restricted to the colonial settlers, who embody a growing metropolitan monopoly over knowledge and culture. They zealously discredit traditional authority and spellbind the natives with their powerful metropolitan sciences. Later, a few natives are absorbed into the professional layer. The handful of local nurses and doctors, thoroughly inculcated with the values of a metropolitan education, prove generally to be pliant intermediaries and willing collaborators of the colonial regime.

The most dramatic means by which medicine creates new social relations is through the differential provision of services. In Morocco, the colonial regime set up a medical system with widely varying services in a conscious effort to promote new social divisions. These divisions were deemed necessary for governance and for profitable colonial production. Divide-and-rule policies were the basis of separate services for Europeans, Moroccan Jews, and Moroccan Muslims. This ethnic segmentation overlapped with class-based distinctions. The result was high-quality care for settlers, officials, army officers, and Moroccan notables; poor to moderate care for Moroccan urban wage workers, small shopkeepers, and petty bureaucrats; and a rudimentary to nonexistent care for the urban unemployed and the peasant masses in the countryside.

The level of medical care was not static, but changed from time to time in response to changing labor force requirements. When plagues or economic expansion caused labor shortages, the budgets for mass medical services were increased; conversely, when the labor supply was overabundant due to depressions or previous medical successes, health budgets were pared down. After independence, the French-sponsored neocolonial health service abolished the odious ethnic separation, but the differential provision of health care, based on the requirements of governance and production, remained in force.

American overseas medical policy likewise favors a class-based health approach. Heavy American support for medical technology reinforces a hospital-centered urban medicine which serves primarily the most privileged elements of society. American training programs for physicians extend specialization and private practice, the high fees for which exclude all but the wealthy few. While fostering quality medical enclaves for the local intermediaries of American power, American policy has retarded the development of decent health care for the masses. The labor supply in these countries is so far in excess of capital's current requirements that millions of unemployed threaten the stability of the social order; American policy has aimed to reduce these unruly population "surpluses." Aid programs have enforced efficiency budgeting, fiscal austerity, and population control in medical planning. Many client regimes have thus curtailed their already modest mass medical programs, substituting birth control efforts instead.[18]

CONTRADICTIONS OF IMPERIALIST MEDICINE

Imperialist medicine promotes political control, social inequality, and exploitation, but it also contains many contradictions. It promotes new forms of consciousness, social structure, and political action that threaten the foundations of the imperialist social order.

In the realm of ideas, medicine is not all mystification. It fosters rationality, scientific thought and optimism. Its promise of prolonged life and vastly improved health, however imperfectly

realized, helps to break the bond of religious fatalism that has kept the peasant masses resigned to millennial misery. It opens up hope and even expectation of a world controlled by human will and human need. In short, it lays the groundwork for a revolutionary approach to the human condition, which medical diplomacy, espionage, and propaganda find difficulty containing.

Medicine also promotes the development of a class of wage workers. As this colonial proletariat passes from the waiting lines of the rural infirmary to the work gangs of the colonial mines and factories, it gains in collective experience, organization, and self-confidence. Rebelling against the shoddy health services as against the harsh bosses at the point of production, these workers formed the backbone of the independent party in the Moroccan struggle against colonialism. By their attacks on colonial doctors and infirmaries, they signalled an end to the passive acceptance of medical authority and of colonial authority as well. In fact, the fight for national liberation may be seen as a workers' fight for health in the broadest and most profound sense.

Although the Moroccan struggle for independence gained formal political autonomy, its most radical tendencies were defeated and colonial medicine remained intact. But the historical process continued. By helping to call into being an ever larger working class, medicine prepared the ground for yet another stage in the struggle for health. The postcolonial workers' parties—more revolutionary than their nationalist forebears—now insist that life and health are the just rights of all. The doctors and health authorities are righteously indignant at such "impossible" demands. But they fail to realize that imperialist medicine contributes to its own demise.

NOTES

1. The imperialist period begins about the 1870s. At that time, the major capitalist interests of the metropolitan countries—mainly Britian, France, Germany, and the United States—faced reduced opportunities for accumulation at home due to a sharp decline in the rate of profit. They thus embarked on a worldwide quest for new accumulation. Dividing up the globe into imperial spheres of inter-

est, the metropolitan capitalists rapidly established lucrative mines and plantations in the most remote regions and swamped distant and previously localized markets with the produce of metropolitan factories. A world division of labor was thus established in which the markets, labor power, and natural resources of the colonial peripheries were subordinated to the interests of the financiers and manufacturers of the metropolitan centers. This arrangement continues, with few modifications, into the present period. Cf. Walter Rodney, *How Europe Underdeveloped Africa* (Washington, D.C.: Howard University Press, 1974).

2. This is essentially the definition proposed by the World Health Organization.

3. The theoretical foundation of this article and the data on Morocco are based on the author's "Professionals and Politics in Morocco: A Historical Study of the Mediation of Power and the Creation of Ideology in the Context of European Imperialism" (Ph.D. diss., Department of Politics, New York University). In order to simplify the references, we refer the reader who may wish sources on Morocco to the dissertation, esp. pp. 101–30, 166–76 and 318–35. We should also note here that the sections in this paper on medicine and American imperialism are less fully developed than those on Morocco and are intended primarily to suggest likely parallels to the Moroccan experience.

4. We refer here to grants and loans of USAID for the period 1965 through 1974. The total was $1,152.2 million; $529.7 million for "health" projects and $622.5 million for "population and family planning" projects. A more global figure, including private philanthropy and other government agencies, would obviously be much higher.

5. "Vietnam—A Medical Victory at Least?" *Medical World News*, June 2, 1975, p. 33. These are U. S. government estimates and doubtless conservative.

6. See Bertrand Russell Peace Foundation, *The Silent Slaughter: The Role of the United States in the Indonesian Massacre* (New York: 1966); Norman Gall, "Guatemalan Slaughter," *New York Review of Books* (May 1971); "Chile," *NACLA's Latin American and Empire Report* 8, no. 5 (May–June 1974).

7. This point is developed at length in a forthcoming book by Sol Yurick and Steve Kandell tentatively titled *Food, Energy, and Genocide*. Other authors who have alluded to the same process are Barry Commoner and René Dumont.

8. See Alfred W. McCoy, *The Politics of Heroin in Southeast Asia* (New York, 1972).

9. The Count of Saint-Aulaire, as quoted in Maroc Médical, *Lyautey et le Médecin* (Casablanca, 1954), p. 13.

10. *The Untapped Resource: Medicine and Diplomacy* (Maryknoll, 1971), pp. 3–4. For a more extended treatment on the same subject, see Cahill's article, "Medicine and Diplomacy in the Tropics," *New York Journal of Medicine* 67 (1967): 2229–38. We might note that American diplomacy has also made use of local doctors and their access to persons in high places. Philip Agee, in his most recent book, *Inside the Company: CIA Diary*, has reported one such case. It seems that the agency employed a Colombian doctor named Ovalle who was the personal physician of Equadorian President Velasco Ibarra. Ovalle communicated weekly with the CIA, passing along intimate details of his client's personal and official life.

11. Leonard R. Friedman, "American Medicine as a Military-Political Weapon," *Military Medicine* 131, no. 10 (October 1966): 1273–77.

12. Spurgeon Neel, "The Medical Role in Army Stability Operations," *Military Medicine* 132, no. 8 (August 1967): 605–8.

13. "The War We Can Win," in Cahill, *The Untapped Resource*, p. 104. Carey is currently governor of the state of New York and Cahill is his chief medical advisor.

14. "Medicine at War—II," *New York Times*, May 29, 1966, p. 59.

15. Howard A. Rusk, "Vietnam Medicine—I," *New York Times*, October 1, 1967, p. 80.

16. From interviews with officials of World Health Organization. USAID unfortunately does not publish a report on its "health" aid.

17. See William Barclay et al., "Population Control in the Third World," *NACLA Newsletter* 4, no. 8 (December 1970).

18. The clear preponderance of population control monies in U.S. medical aid is a clear indication of this priority. The United States government, in conjunction with the World Bank, has virtually imposed a shift from mass medicine to "family planning" in dozens of countries including India, Brazil, the Philippines, Morocco, and the Dominican Republic.

ADDITIONAL REFERENCES

Louis-Paul Aujoulat. *Santé et dévelopment en Afrique*. Paris: Armand Colin, 1969.

Frantz Fanon. "Medicine and Colonialism," in *Studies in a Dying*

Colonialism. New York: Grove Press, 1967. Reprinted in this volume.

Howard A. Levy. "Bringing the War Back Home," *Health-PAC Bulletin* (April 1970): 1–8.

James A. Paul. "L'organisation de la santé et les médecins après l'indépendence,' *Lamalif* (Casablanca), no. 69 (March 1975): 18–26.

H. M. Singer. "Health as an Instrument of Foregn Policy," *Congressional Record*, February 19, 1968, p. E-870.

HOWARD LEVY
THE MILITARY MEDICINEMEN

Healers and warriors have usually lived in comfortable symbiosis. Physicians follow the exigencies of the war machines they serve—as a wheel turns in response to a drive shaft. Different types of wars have elicited different kinds of responses from physicians, but, after all was said, the end result was the same— the healers served the masters of war well.

It has been claimed that physicians serve in an apolitical capacity during wartime—that they only treat the sick and wounded. This claim is surely specious. In conventional wars (as in the War of 1812), doctors treated primarily their own troops, and, in so doing, strengthened their army's fighting force, which, in turn, was tantamount to offering political support for the mission which that army was pursuing.

In other wars, fought on territory which was medically inhospitable to nonindigenous troops, physicians sought to conquer the endemic diseases which often took a larger toll of soldiers than did militarily-inflicted injuries. Thus, in tropical and semi-tropical theaters of war, physicians conquered malaria and typhoid. In such instances, a definite fallout of the doctor's role was the improved health of civilians. However, this effect was incidental to the physician's primary job—the protection of the lives and bodies of his own troops.

As wars moved into the nuclear age, physicians were prepared to deal with the impossible task of developing medical defenses against nuclear warfare. Though humanitarian physicians might have thought a ban on nuclear war to be the ultimate cure for the destruction of human life by nuclear weapons, military physicians

preferred to develop schemes for the treatment of mass casualties.

Finally, when "people's wars of liberation" became the targets of military strategists, medicine again trailed along meekly behind its master and developed techniques to forestall, and if that was unsuccessful to win, wars in which the entire people of a nation became the enemy. At this juncture, not only were doctors asked to care for the troops of a combatant nation, but they were called upon to placate, tranquilize, and quell enemy insurgency—medicine was quietly adapted to political counterinsurgency.

From time to time healers have reflected upon the inconsistency between healing and killing. Louis Pasteur said:

> Two opposing laws seem to me in contest. The one law of blood and death, opening out each day new modes of destruction, forces nations to be always ready for battle. The other, a law of peace, work, and health, whose only aim is to deliver man from the calamities which beset him. The one seeks violent conquests, the other the relief of mankind. The one places a single life above victories, the other sacrifices hundreds of thousands of lives. Which of these two laws will prevail, only God knows. But of this we may be sure, that science, in obeying the law of humanity, will always labor to enlarge the frontiers of life.

Like Pasteur, physicians have always, despite their occasional qualms, proudly served their countrymen in times of war. Historical trends, dating back at least to the sixteenth century, have been to create the concept of "medicine" as "international," in the abstract, while still recognizing that physicians themselves are first citizens of their own nation and only second citizens of the world. Physicians have therefore been expected to choose sides during wars. They have been expected to strengthen the fighting reserve of the army of which they are a part. In the words of *U.S. Army Field Manual 8-10*:

> The Army Medical Service is a supporting service of the combat elements of the Army primarily concerned with the maintenance of the health and fighting efficiency of the troops. The mission of the medical service in a theater of operations is to conserve manpower by recommending, and providing technical supervision of the implementation of, measures for safeguarding the health of the troops,

effective medical care, and early return to duty; and to contribute directly to the military effort by providing adequate medical treatment and rapid, orderly evacuation for the sick and wounded.

Of course, when the broader, more idealistic concepts of international medicine have not interfered with military operations, there has been an increasing realization that they can and should be invoked during wars, to minimize the brutality of the conflict. Thus as early as sixteenth-century Switzerland, during the wars between the cantons, the return of POW's and the wounded was permitted. Throughout the nineteenth and twentieth centuries these conventions have been strengthened to the point where, in theory at least, the doctor and corpsman and military nurse are not to be thought of as combat soldiers. They are, once again in theory, not a party to war and are therefore granted immunity from attack. It should, however, be noted that these "humanistic" conventions serve the purpose primarily of insuring the all-important existence of a medical presence for contesting armies. And, once again, as *Army Field Manual 8-10* makes clear, this must be so in order to "contribute to the success of the military effort."

Thus the thrust of ethical developments concerning the physician and war has been double: on the one hand, medical skills, *per se*, ought to be utilized in accordance with international humanitarian ideals; on the other, the physician as a man owes his allegiance to his nation and must therefore maintain the fighting efficiency of the troops which are under his care. Of course, it was bound to happen that some physicians would note the apparent contradictory directions of this development. Dr. John A. Ryle, then Regius Professor of Physics at the University of Cambridge, had this to say about the physician, idealistic ethics, and war:

> It is an arresting, if at present a fantastic thought, that the medical profession which is more international than any other, could, if well coordinated, of its own initiative put a stop to war, or at least increase its uncertainties, and temper its aims considerably so as to give pause to the most bellicose of governments. It is everywhere a recognized and humane principle that prevention should be preferred to cure. By withholding service from the Armed Forces be-

fore and during war, by declining to examine and innoculate re-
cruits, by refusing sanitary advice and the training and command of
ambulances, clearing stations, medical transport, and hospitals, the
doctors could so cripple the efficiency of the staff and aggravate the
difficulties of campaign and so damage the morale of the troops that
war would become almost unthinkable. Action of this kind would
also produce profound effect on the popular imagination. In such
refusal of service . . . there would be no inhumanity which
medicine at present sanctions and prolongs.

Ryle, however, in a concluding sentence, recognized, at least
intuitively, the fallacy of his reasoning when he wrote, "But let
the dream pass and fantasy make room for facts." The facts,
indeed, are that so international a medical community as would
be required to make Ryle's dream a reality does not exist. Nor
could one survive in a politically and economically splintered
world body. It is far from reasonable to assume that class
privileged physicians of even a single nation would unite in any
moral action antithetical to their class interest.

Still, in the United States the armed forces have had, until
relatively recently, a respectful attitude toward the underlying
humanitarian ethical considerations of medicine as an international healing agent. Medicine has been treated in wartime in a
comparatively apolitical manner. In a narrow sense the doctor's
efforts on behalf of and allegiance to one fighting force in preference to the opposing army functioned tactically to strengthen
that side. The political consequences of serving in such a partisan
role surely cannot be ignored. But what other options could be
offered to allow the doctor to share in his nation's political destiny? At the same time, a brief review of U.S. military medicine
illustrates that American physicians, while until very recently,
willingly sharing their nation's historic role, have also preserved
the philosophical ideal of medicine as an agent of international
good will.

It is of striking importance that during the American Revolution of 1776, while some doctors served as military physicians
(e.g., Benjamin Rush), other American doctor-revolutionists
eagerly sought the high ground of the battlefield. One hundred
eighty years before Che Guevara, these humanists acted, as their

South American professional kinsman did later, militarily to broaden the freedom and well-being of their countrymen. The following doctors became revolutionary heroes performing not as battlefield surgeons, but rather as military leaders: Major-Generals Joseph Warren (killed at the Battle of Bunker Hill), Oliver Prescott, John Brooks, John Thomas, Arthur St. Clair; Brigadier Generals Hugh Mercer, Edward Hand, and William Irvine. It is of interest that two physicians, James McHenry and William Eustis, ultimately became secretaries of war of the fledgling nation.

After winning the American war of national liberation, the American army formally developed a well-defined medical corps. In subsequent wars, up until the Vietnam war, American military physicians served not as military tacticians and commanders, but as doctors in support of their troops. This was the case in the Indian wars, the War of 1812, and the Mexican War. In a limited sense medicine could be said to have played a "neutral" role—it was limited to the treatment and care of wounded men on either side. It was not used directly in itself as a political weapon.

This "neutrality" was temporarily breached during the American Civil War. The Union army's blockade of needed drugs and supplies was used to weaken not only the Confederate army but the people of the Confederacy as a whole. The results of the blockade were serious indeed, and were especially serious for Union prisoners of war. Here medicine was used tactically in a negative manner as an instrument of war policy and not merely indirectly in support of a fighting army.

Medicine again resumed a supportive role in the Spanish-American War of 1898. But new conditions of warfare beyond what are now the continental limits of the United States necessitated that this medical support assume new duties and responsibilities. With the Spanish-American War, the construction of the militarily and commercially strategic Panama Canal, and the deployment of the "Army of Pacification" into Cuba in 1906, diseases such as typhoid and yellow fever became more serious depleters of military strength than were battlefield casualties. And physician-soldiers such as Walter Reed and William Crawford Gorgas established their military and medical reputations in suc-

cessfully combating these diseases. In so doing, they preserved the fighting strength of American troops and thus were clearly prime agents of what had become by 1898 a consciously imperialistic American foreign policy. Still, agents though they were, their use of medicine was nonetheless militarily supportive and not directly offensive. Typhoid and yellow fever were controlled in parts of Latin America, not to convince the indigenous inhabitants of the justice of American militarism, but merely to insure the success of imperialist expansion by preventing the death of thousands of American soldiers and civilians from diseases which were endemic to these parts of the world. For example, the deaths of 22,000 Frenchmen from "Yellow Jack" prevented their building the Panama Canal. Reed's investigations, which linked this disease to the mosquito, and the subsequent practical application of this discovery by Gorgas, together with the American military intervention in Panama, provided the margin of safety which permitted the American Panama Canal effort to succeed where the French had previously failed, and thus permitted the United States a major imperialist expansion into Central America.

In World War I, battlefield casualties exceeded deaths from natural diseases. As a consequence, important innovations in the care of battlefield injuries were pursued and practiced. The supportive role of the medical corps on the battlefield was reflected by the fact that the death rate of the medical corpsmen was higher than the death rates, respectively, of Aviation, Cavalry, Engineers, Ordnance, and Quarter-Master Corps. Only Infantry, Artillery, Tanks, and Signal Corps had higher casualty rates.

In World War II, the motto of the Medical Field Service School was "To Conserve Fighting Strength." And indeed this had been the operative motif of the Army Medical Corps in all wars since the Revolutionary War up until the time of the war in Vietnam.

In Vietnam, an important departure from this heretofore sole mission was clearly in evidence. The Medical Corps still had as its primary mission the preservation of the life and well-being of American troops, but now assumed, in addition, a direct political role. Before turning to the evidence as it manifests itself fully in

Vietnam, we should first trace the theoretical development of this new role.

The genesis of America's conscious, positive utilization of medicine as a political weapon of counterinsurgency actually began in the early twentieth century but was little appreciated at the time and was to remain a practically unknown phenomenon until after World War II. But in 1902, Col. Leonard Wood, M.D., was dispatched to the provinces of the Moros in the Philippines. Wood had previously served as part of an American military pacification team in Cuba. (Cuba had been "liberated" from Spain by the United States in the midst of a Cuban war of national liberation against Spain. The United States then succeeded, where Spain had failed, in pacifying the country by force.)

It was Wood's mission in the Philippines to pacify the imminent insurgency of the islands' mistreated Moslem population. During his first Philippine mission, Wood engaged the Nomasites Missionaries and soldiers in teaching the Moslems to read. After a fourteen-year absence, Wood returned to the Philippines for a second tour in 1921, only to find that his efforts at "nation building" were in a state of disarray. Wood and his successor, Frank McCoy, consciously used public health measures, such as the implementation of sanitary programs, to pacify various potential insurgent ethnic groups. Wood's program of civic action was the seminal idea which was later to bloom into the Special Forces and the Peace Corps. But it was not until after World War II that medicine as a counterinsurgency weapon was attempted again in a systematic way through direct intervention of America's military forces.

At the end of World War II Supreme Commander General Douglas MacArthur's first directive to the Japanese people was a "Bill of Rights" issued on October 4, 1945. As a part of that postwar pacification program, MacArthur instructed the American occupying army to institute a wide array of public health measures. Brigadier General Crawford F. Sams developed a program in which 80 million Japanese were vaccinated against smallpox. Other programs were directed against scabies, typhus, TB, dysentery, and cholera.

Under the Marshall Plan similar programs were developed for

the war-devastated nations of Europe with their intent being, in large part, the rebuilding of nations whose governments would be pliable and friendly to the interests of the United States. Medicine was a small, though not insignificant, part of that effort. But where civic action programs faltered, as in post-World War II Italy and Greece, military support was forthcoming. The ruling principle was to forestall the democratic installation of Communist governments at any cost. The combination of economic and medical assistance with military support was successful, at least for the time being.

It should be observed that following World War II, large areas of Europe and Japan lay in ruins. To rehabilitate these nations could be thought of as an elementary humanitarian requirement. However, a great deal of historical evidence supports the contention that United States support for the rebuilding of Japan and Western Europe was based, first, upon political need, and only second was in response to human need.

Soon after the conclusion of World War II the United States became immersed in the chilly waters of the Cold War. And a nuclear deterrence mentality permeated foreign policy. For most of the 1950s military publications and military medical journals, when they concerned themselves with politics at all, were principally concerned with aspects of medical defense against nuclear attack. But it should not be imagined that the previous instances of at least temporarily successful counterinsurgency pacification programs had been entirely forgotten.

The spirit of medical pacification was resurrected in September 1957, when President Eisenhower announced his "People-to-People Program." He said, "All of us thoroughly believe the people themselves want to be friends and it is as much the duty of professional military officers to enhance and help develop that feeling of friendliness of people as to be capable of defense in case of attack." A few years later, that innocuous-sounding sentence was to become the foundation for America's present counterinsurgency program.

The March 1961 issue of *Army*, the monthly magazine of the Association of the U.S. Army, heralded a new stage of United States militarism. (*Army's* articles and themes are often later

picked up by such popular magazines as *Readers' Digest*.) A story in that issue launched what was to prove to be a major propaganda and educational program aimed at convincing the American people that counterinsurgency was the best designed tactic to defend U.S. economic and political interests. And what better way to pave the way for this switch of emphasis than to publish serially Che Guevara's *Manual of Guerrilla Warfare*?

In June 1961 *Army* devoted its cover story to a then little-known branch of the army—the Special Forces. The story was titled, "Special Forces—What They Are." Article followed upon article on the new tactic of counterinsurgency. One by George V. Tanham was titled, "Wars Without Guns." Tanham had been a former Associate Director of Provincial Operations in the Agency for International Development (AID). His office was in Saigon.

The switch in propaganda emphasis from nuclear brinksmanship to counterinsurgency was dramatic, although one can be sure that the actual policy was planned well in advance. The Special Forces had, in fact, been formed in 1952. During the Korean War they served behind the lines, through not in a medical role. It was not, however, until after the election of John F. Kennedy that the Special Forces were made an object of adulation. And, under Kennedy, the Special Forces medical program probably was originated in early 1962.

If *Army* was used as the vehicle to launch the U.S. Military's new propaganda offensive in March 1961, *Military Medicine*, an official publication of the Association of Military Surgeons, was not far behind. In April 1961 *Military Medicine* carried an article titled, "The Role of the Army Medical Service in 'America's People-to-People Program' " written by Lt. General Leonard D. Heaton, M.D., the Surgeon General of the U.S. Army. Heaton's takeoff point was Eisenhower's People-to-People program, but his vision went far beyond. In concluding his article, Heaton wrote: "In offering our medical skills . . . we can surely receive more than we give [in terms of preventing the spread of Communism]."

Other articles followed quickly on the heels of Heaton's opening salvo. Some attempted to show that counterinsurgency was but a continuation of the post-World War II European and Eastern Asian reconstruction program. The link between programs

such as the Marshall Plan and active counterinsurgency for the "undeveloped" parts of the world was Korea. In an article titled, "International Medicine" (January 1962), Brigadier General Howard W. Doan, Deputy Surgeon General of the Army, alluded to the Korean experience. Quoting the previous Chief of the Military Medical Services in Korea, Doan wrote, "By choosing kindness, charity and usefulness, U.S. military citizens in Korea and in other countries too have done much to reveal to the less fortunate world citizen the fruits of the principles on which our God-fearing nation was established. Citizens can be grateful for the contribution our armed forces have made worldwide to the human values of Christianity and democracy." He then equated the Army Military Medical Service with "Military Missionary Medical Work," and, as if to underscore the point, later included the Agency for International Development, Albert Schweitzer, and Dr. Tom Dooley as part of America's new anticommunist crusade.

By October 1966 *Military Medicine* was prepared to begin shedding the euphemisms and presented an article, "American Medicine as a Military-Political Weapon," by Captain Leonard R. Friedman, a psychiatrist stationed with the Special Forces at the JFK Special Warfare Center, Fort Bragg. The thrust of the article was that

> future American policy might well express itself in the health, education and welfare of all Vietnamese minorities and ethnic groups. Such an effort might be directed both toward the minorities and toward the Central Government, in an effort to create and maintain a bond of mutual trust between divergent cultures, through medicine.

Thus a contribution might be made "to a solution of the South Vietnamese insurgency."

The following month's issue of *Military Medicine* carried an article by the Surgeon General of the Air Force, R. L. Bohannon, M.D. General Bohannon attempted to give legitimacy to the newly rediscovered political use of medicine by quoting Sir William Osler. Osler, it seems, addressed the 1894 graduating class of the Army Medical School and reminded the recent grad-

uates that farflung military posts ("Florida Keys to Montana, from Maine to Southern California") can be used to study a diversity of morbid conditions. Osler was especially impressed by the possibilities in Indian territories, and from that General Bohannon concluded that Osler's remarks could be construed as "an early reference to medical civic action, now as you know, a most important factor in the second facet [the pacification program] of the war in South Vietnam."

By February 1967, literary and historical reserve were finally thrown to the wind. *Military Medicine* reprinted a speech in which General Heaton alluded to General MacArthur—but the allusion wasn't to the MacArthur who pacified postwar Japan with public health measures. Rather, Heaton referred to the MacArthur who said, "The soldier . . . is required to practice the greatest act of religious training—sacrifice." Medicine, Heaton continued, is "today, more than ever before, inescapably inwoven in our foreign policy." Medicine provides "a secure route to a greater appreciation of our peaceful intentions." The mode, the creed, the way of life of the Army Medical Service is "Duty, Honor, Country. . . . God Bless Them." So closed General Heaton.

Perhaps the definitive statement regarding the U.S. army's new face of medicine was written in August 1967 by Col. Spurgeon Neel. Neel, a doctor, was the Surgeon of the United States Military Assistance Command, Vietnam. Neel's article clearly spelled out the ABCs of medical counterinsurgency. His outline bears study, since it is the operative model not merely for the U.S. army in Vietnam but also for the Special Forces, AID, and Peace Corps in a score of countries all over the world. Neel proceeds as follows:

Point 1: "Medical stability operations concentrate on the pre-insurgency phase—to produce maximum results with minimum resource investment."

Point 2: The program must provide "medical treatment for immediate impact, and preventive medicine projects to produce short-term improvement."

Point 3: Medicine is an ideal civic action program because its "humanitarian aspects . . . can be raised above the level of

political turbulence." It provides an "apolitical avenue through which favorable influence may be maintained." And it "provides immediate high-impact communication."

Point 4: The program must be a coordinated effort of "the country team." The country team includes the U.S. army, Green Berets, USAID, and the ambassador to the country in question.

Point 5: As in one of the Vietnam medical programs, a key goal is the "maintenance of the favorable image of the Central Government of Vietnam [or Laos, Thailand, Dominican Republic, Guatemala, etc.] and of the U.S. in the minds of the general population."

Point 6: To assist in reaching this goal in Vietnam, "U.S. military hospitals admit selected Vietnamese civilians for 'high impact' surgical procedures." This phase of the program concentrates on children who suffer from major disfiguring illnesses such as "harelips, burn contractures, orthopedic deformities. . . . The psychological impact on the inhabitants of the village to which the restored patient is returned is tremendous."

Neel's outline was brought up to date and slightly amplified in May 1968 by Lt. Col. Charles R. Webb, M.D. Interestingly enough, Webb pointed out that the term "counterinsurgency" was no longer in vogue and had been replaced by the phrase "Internal Defense and Development (ID/D)." Webb also details newer facets of medical counterinsurgency operations. He states, "Another important facet of medicine in ID/D involves the denial of medical resources to the insurgents." Further, Webb assures us that "much valuable intelligence can be gathered from a local medical system. People under treatment are frequently very cooperative in revealing information about the guerrilla force." We've come a long way from Sir William Osler.

Vietnam has been the laboratory in which Americans experiment with medical counterinsurgency technics. What have been the results to date? South Vietnam, with a population of about 17 million, has available between four hundred and five hundred indigenous physicians. In most provinces, the two or three doctors live in the provincial capital and rarely venture out to the outlying countryside. Hospitals are scarce, many having been built in the nineteenth century and often not being equipped

with running water. Overcrowding and poor sanitary facilities within the hospitals are the rule, with two or three patients frequently sharing a single bed.

Cholera and plague are prevalent in South Vietnam. And, in areas of the country where U.S. servicemen are concentrated, syphilis and gonorrhea rates reach epidemic proportions. Other health problems include TB, sanitation, and poor water supply. The prevalence of these diseases and problems may have something to do with the fact that the Saigon government devotes only 1 percent of its national budget to medical expenses. This represents the lowest such percentage in the world. North Vietnam, by contrast, has eliminated plague, cholera, and dengue-like diseases. According to WHO, North Vietnam's health services "give the impression of a resolute endeavor to provide a comprehensive health service according to a national health plan which is consistent with national aspirations, needs, and resources."

Meanwhile, back in South Vietnam an army physician is probably still experiencing most of the difficulties which Capt. Daniel White wrote about in 1968:

All medicine must be given on a day-to-day basis because many patients cannot be relied upon to take their medication as prescribed. . . . A significant number [of patients] are never seen again after their initial visit. . . . Resistance is encountered frequently when consent for surgery is sought.

Dr. White's experience recalls the words of another doctor, Frantz Fanon, the Algerian psychiatrist revolutionist. Fanon reported that in French colonial Algeria the patients also resisted hospitalization, surgery, medication. "Accepting the medicine," Fanon explains, "is admitting . . . the validity of Western technique. It is demonstrating one's confidence in the foreigner's medical science." After the victory of the revolution these problems were resolved because medical care was no longer dispensed by an enemy of the people and a doctor "was no longer 'the doctor,' but 'our' doctor." Fanon concludes, "The people who take their destiny into their own hands assimilate the most modern forms of technology at an extraordinary rate."

But the United States is still playing at the medical missionary

game. And the game itself is but a facade shielding the role of medicine as an arm of American foreign policy. Unlike the traditional political impact which the military physician always had when concerning himself primarily with the medical needs of his own troops, the entire concept of medicine as an entity has become politicized. The political effects of the Internal Defense and Development physician are no longer incidental or indirect, they are now his sole preoccupation, or rather his raison d'être.